Case Studies in Breastfeeding

Related Titles from Jones and Bartlett

Reclaiming Breastfeeding for the United States: Protection, Promotion, and Support, Cadwell

Maternal and Infant Assessment for Breastfeeding and Human Lactation: A Guide for the Practitioner, Cadwell/Turner-Maffei/O'Connor/Blair

Impact of Birthing Practices on Breastfeeding: Protecting the Mother and Baby Continuum, Kroeger

Counseling the Nursing Mother: A Lactation Consultant's Guide, Third Edition, Lauwers/Shinskie

Pocket Guide for Counseling the Nursing Mother, Shinskie/Lauwers

Breastfeeding and Human Lactation, Second Edition, Riordan/Auerbach

Pocket Guide to Breastfeeding and Human Lactation, Second Edition, Riordan/Auerbach

The Lactation Consultant in Private Practice: The ABCs of Getting Started, Smith

Coach's Notebook: Games and Strategies for Lactation Education, Smith

World Headquarters
Jones and Bartlett Publishers
40 Tall Pine Drive
Sudbury, MA 01776
978-443-5000
info@jbpub.com
www.jbpub.com

Jones and Bartlett Publishers Canada
2406 Nikanna Road
Mississauga, ON L5C 2W6
CANADA

Jones and Bartlett Publishers International
Barb House, Barb Mews
London W6 7PA
UK

Copyright © 2004 by Jones and Bartlett Publishers, Inc.

Library of Congress Cataloging-in-Publication Data

Cadwell, Karin.
    Case studies in breastfeeding : problem-solving skills & strategies / Karin Cadwell, Cynthia Turner-Maffei.
        p. cm.
    Includes bibliographical references and index.
    ISBN 0-7637-2600-1
        1. Breast feeding—Case studies. 2. Breast feeding—Complications—Case studies. I. Turner-Maffei, Cynthia. II. Title.

    RJ216.C228 2003
    613.2'69—dc21

                                                                2003054347

Acquisitions Editor: Penny M. Glynn
Production Manager: Amy Rose
Associate Production Editor: Jenny L. McIsaac
Editorial Assistant: Amy Sibley
Associate Marketing Manager: Joy Stark-Vancs
Marketing Associate: Elizabeth Waterfall
Manufacturing Buyer: Amy Bacus
Cover Design: Kristin E. Ohlin
Interior Design: Dartmouth Publishing, Inc.
Composition: GEX, Inc.
Printing and Binding: Malloy Inc.
Cover Printing: Malloy Inc.

Printed in the United States of America
07 06 05   10 9 8 7 6 5 4 3 2

Case Studies in Breastfeeding

Problem-Solving Skills & Strategies

KARIN CADWELL, PhD, RN, IBCLC

CYNTHIA TURNER-MAFFEI, MA, IBCLC

JONES AND BARTLETT PUBLISHERS
Sudbury, Massachusetts
BOSTON   TORONTO   LONDON   SINGAPORE

Table of Contents

Foreword

Kajsa Drimdyr, PhD

> *Stories are more than a celebration of practice; they are an essential part of the practice to be celebrated.*
>
> —JULIAN ORR, WORK PRACTICE
> ANTHROPOLOGIST (1945–)

Many professions and professionals rely on stories. Early childhood educators use stories, myths, and legends as part of their curricula in order to model appropriate and inappropriate behavior for the children they teach. Researchers in the field of Artificial Intelligence use the stories and scripts of human behavior gleaned from Cognitive Psychology to learn how to elicit the appropriate (human) response of a computer as they develop programs. The field of Organizational Development emphasizes the central importance of revealing workplace stories, history, and corporate beliefs as a key aspect of organizational culture.

Stories and their use in professional development have been investigated. Julian Orr[1] wondered about the role of stories in the development and maintenance of proficiency in the work force. He studied copier repair technicians, experts and novices, who had received classroom and hands-on training in order to work on copiers placed in organizations.

Orr noticed that copier repair technicians often work in isolation. They are considered to be a peripheral or perhaps marginal part of the corporation by management. He noticed that they can tell if something is not working properly, but don't know whether that contributes to the designated problem. The technicians use the narrative of their

---

[1] Orr, Julian E. *Talking about Machines: an ethnography of a modern job*. IRL Press Cornell, New York: 1996.

customers to look for absences, to try to determine what is wrong and why. They need to use the skills of ear, hand, and eye—noting how something sounds, or a non-verbal sense of correctness to determine the diagnosis. There are questions about the definition of the work that they do—differences according to the corporations, employers, and the technicians themselves. There are questions about the source of the authoritative knowledge, as well as about where that knowledge is stored and preserved.

The style of work of copier repair technicians may not seem to be directly related to that of lactation professionals. But some of the similarities seem striking. Orr offers the view he observed of their situation:

> *"Understanding the problem determines what is to be done about it, but understanding is created from an assortment of information that does not necessarily point to a single diagnosis. The practice of diagnosis is done through narrative, and both diagnosis and process are preserved and circulated among the technicians through war stories, anecdotes of their experiences."* *(Orr, p. 104)*

Julian Orr's research into the work practice of copier repair personnel revealed their use of story. He found a culture of "war stories" to bring novices up to speed and to share information about solving difficult and unusual cases. These stories formed a vital core of the work education of the technicians—one that is intangible, and therefore easily lost with changes to management or reorganization.

Starting with the assumption that the technicians understand the basic concepts related to the machine, they must take in "an assortment of information" and sort through it, using stories and discussion, to determine a diagnosis, at which point the stories are shared with others to help with future problem solving. These war stories are especially important when "no clear formulation of the problem is emerging from the welter of facts".

What is the role of story to a lactation professional? In this often isolated profession, the sharing of stories is central and essential. They represent a way of sorting through information gathered—from the mother, from the baby, from other health professionals—in order to determine the diagnosis. They also represent an important, often invisible, archive of knowledge to help with future problem solving. These intangible elements are most often shared informally—with colleagues or to add color to a presentation—and then are lost. It is vital to preserve and share the experiences and stories of the practitioners in the field in order to grow a professional knowledge base.

The stories of a profession bridge the gap between theory and practice. Ingela Josefson's[2] research of newly qualified nurses in relation to experienced nurses demonstrates the importance of integrating their theoretical knowledge with practical experience. Learned information, from a classroom or book, represents an important starting point for gaining knowledge. But as this knowledge is placed in a context, a specific story, it grows and evolves to apply to the specific challenges of the situation. Jean Lave[3], who focuses on the ideas of context, and situating information in order to make sense of it, explains that "knowledge always undergoes construction and transformation in use." The stories of lactation cases and their solutions, the experiences of experts, need to be shared with others in the profession to develop and strengthen a shared knowledge base.

Karin Cadwell and Cynthia Turner-Maffei have, in this volume, made a significant contribution to the development of lactation consulting as a profession as they bring forward the stories and diagnosis that experts can, and should, share with novices and other experts in the field. They are bringing the knowledge into the context of the work. This book represents an important step to both bringing the stories of a profession to novices, and to sharing information about solving difficult and unusual cases among experts.

---

[2] Josefson, Ingela. "Language and Experience" in Bo Göranzon and Magnus Florin (eds). *Artificial Intelligence, Culture and Language*. Springer Verlag, London: 1990.

[3] Lave, Jean "The practice of learning" in Jean Lave and Seth Chaiklin (eds). *Understanding Practice: Perspectives on activity and context*. Cambridge University Press, Cambridge: 1996.

Acknowledgements

We gratefully acknowledge the National Gallery of London, England for giving us permission to use the beautiful artwork "The Origin of the Milky Way" by Jacopo Tintoretto (1518-1594) on the cover of this book. The scene depicted is that of the Greek God Zeus (Roman name Jupiter) bringing baby Herakles (Hercules) to suckle at the breast of the sleeping Hera (Juno), Zeus's wife. Herakles is the love child of Zeus and Alcmene, a mortal woman. Zeus wants Herakles to receive the milk of a goddess, because it bestows immortal life, and will make Herakles into a god. Zeus anticipates that Hera will not willingly provide her milk to his love child. Therefore, he tries to sneak up on her while she is sleeping. However, foreshadowing his adult strength, the baby Herakles attaches forceably to Hera's breast, awakening her. Hera reacts by pushing the baby off her breast. Her milk spurts forth into the heavens, and creates the stars of what becomes our galaxy, the Milky Way.

We dedicate this book to the growing force of new breastfeeding protectors, supporters, and promoters who we have taught, mentored, and precepted. They are the new stars in our expanding galaxy.

We also gratefully acknowledge the guidance, input, and insight of the many families, breastfeeding advocates, and health care providers with whom we have had the honor of working during our careers. The light shed by these individuals and their stories forms the stars of our personal galaxy, serving as guideposts, lighting the way as we navigate the Milky Way.

Introduction

*To have ideas is to gather flowers; to
think is to weave them into garlands.*

—MME. ANNE SOPHIE SWETCHINE,
AUTHOR (1782–1857)

This book is about weaving garlands. It's about the synthesis of logic,
wisdom, and theory. We have woven these ideas—these garlands—in
order to convey a deeper understanding of how to act and when to act in
accordance with the highest needs of the breastfeeding mother and baby.

The Healthy Children Project's Center for Breastfeeding, with fund-
ing from the United States Department of Health and Human Services,
Public Health Service, Health Resources and Services Administration,
Maternal and Child Health Bureau, investigated the education and
training needs of lactation care providers in 1999 and 2000. In addition
to developing continuing education programs, the faculty of the
Healthy Children Project was also able to initiate bachelors, masters,
and doctoral programs in the field of lactation consulting. These programs are offered in partnership with the Union Institute and University
and have qualified for the accelerated Pathway C of the International
Board of Lactation Consultant Examiners (IBLCE) examination.
Degrees in lactation consulting may serve to enhance the professional

status of those with the IBCLC credential.[1] The Healthy Children Project is invested in educating providers to become interdisciplinary professionals in the field of breastfeeding and human lactation.

Members of an aspiring profession must consider all of the issues involved in rising to full professional status. According to Edgar Schein, writing in his classic book, *Professional Education*, there are three components of professional knowledge:[2]

1. An underlying discipline or basic science component upon which the practice rests or from which it is developed;

   In the interdisciplinary field of lactation, biology, anatomy and physiology, sociology, anthropology, and psychology provide most of the underlying basic science foundation.

2. An applied science or "engineering" component from which many of the diagnostic procedures and problem solutions are derived;

   The Eight Level Lactation Consulting Process™[3] we use in this volume along with our prior book, Maternal and Infant Assessment for Breastfeeding and Human Lactation[4] *are examples of this "engineering" component.*

3. A skills and attitudinal component that concerns the actual performance of services to the client using the underlying basic and applied knowledge.

   In this book we present an "engineering" component, the Eight Levels, and connect it to the skills and attitudinal component through the use of case studies from our practice. Our case studies concern the "actual performance of services to the client," as Schein requires.

---

[1] The International Board of Lactation Consultant Examiners awards the IBCLC credential. For additional information about the IBCLC credential contact IBLCE International Board of Lactation Consultant Examiners, 7309 Arlington Blvd, Suite 300; Falls Church, VA 22042-3215 USA; Phone: 703-560-7330; email: iblce@iblce.org

[2] Schein E. *Professional Education*. New York: McGraw Hill; 1973. p. 43.

[3] The Eight Level Lactation Consulting Process is a trademark of the Healthy Children Project.

[4] Cadwell K, Turner-Maffei C, O'Connor B, Blair A. *Maternal and Infant Assessment for Breastfeeding and Human Lactation: A Guide for the Practitioner*. Sudbury, MA: Jones and Bartlett Publishers; 2002.

> *The universe is made of stories,*
> *not of atoms.*
>
> —MURIEL RUKEYSER,
> POET, BIOGRAPHER (1913–1980)

This is a book of case studies, stories of mothers, babies, and families with whom we have worked. These are memorable cases from which we learned as much as the mother and baby.

Breastfeeding—the English term for the key mammalian interchange of infancy—focuses our attention on the natural process of making and taking milk. Yet, mothers' stories and struggles about feeding belie the "naturalness" of breastfeeding. The process is about so much more than feeding. Other languages have more evocative terms for this interchange. In German, the word for this interchange is *stillen*, which means to calm, to quiet. In Spanish, the word *amamantar* means to mother and protect. The American term *nurse* carries the connotation of breastfeeding, yet this meaning is limited to America. In other English-speaking countries, anyone can "nurse" a baby—it has nothing to do with suckling, but rather with caretaking.

Clinical work in lactation allows us the great privilege of sharing the lived experience of others during a joyful and vulnerable time in their lives. This window into human experience is unique. The family's senses are opened to take in the new family member in their midst. Parents ask themselves: Who is this new baby? What new personality, strengths, character traits have arrived? Who am I in relation to this baby? Will I be a good parent to this child?

All of this questioning and internal reorganizing of the family is done in the context of the enormous crisis/opportunity of birth, and weeks of broken sleep and fatigue. Is it any wonder that their normal polished veneer, the competent face they are used to showing to the outer world, is thin or missing?

> *For all the science that underpins clinical practice,*
> *practitioners and patients make sense of the world by*
> *way of stories.*[5]

---

[5] Elwyn G, Gwyn R. Stories we hear and stories we tell: Analysing talk in clinical practice. *Br Med J*; 318:186–188; 1999.

Telling one's story is an interchange that is, in itself, potentially therapeutic. Listening to a story can provide clinical insight. The process of learning from case studies has been called "narrative based" practice.[6] In our consulting practice, we strive to evoke the story, the present lived experience of the family. We find that when a new mother is inspired to tell us her story, we are able to learn about the organic nature of the problem or problems she seeks to solve. Her narrative helps illustrate the meaning of the problem, its context, and her perspective on the world.

Greenhalgh & Hurwitz write about narrative based clinical practice:

> *The oral tradition of myths and legends, which are continually recreated by word of mouth in successive generations, still features prominently in many non-Western societies and impacts profoundly on the experience of health and illness in these societies. Perhaps it is partly because Western culture has lost its grip on this oral tradition that the skills of listening to, appreciating, and interpreting patients' stories are only rarely upheld as core clinical skills. . . .The core clinical skills of listening, questioning, delineating, marshalling, explaining, and interpreting may provide a way of mediating between the very different worlds of patients and health professionals. Whether these tasks are performed well or badly is likely to have as much influence on the outcome of the illness from the patient's point of view as the more scientific technical aspects of diagnosis or treatment.[7]*

We seek, in our narrative based clinical practice, to understand not just the mother's words, but the feelings behind them, listening with all of our faculties for the surface and deeper meanings of her experience. Although many breastfeeding problems reside in the realm of the baby's mouth position on the surface of the mother's breast, there is almost always a deeper level of questioning from the mother about her ability to adequately "feed" her new baby on the physical, emotional, and spiritual levels. The line between nutrition and nurturing is blurred not only by the similarity in their spelling. In our experience concerns about adequacy of feeding are often tangled up with fears of one's ability to give enough love.

---

[6] Greenhalgh T, Hurwitz B. Narrative based medicine: Why study narrative? *Br Med J*; 318:48–50, 1999.

[7] Greenhalgh & Hurwitz, p. 50.

What we are sharing here is our narrative as told to us by the mother, baby, and other present family members. This is narrative as seen through our lenses, not as directly seen by the family.

Listening is a key skill of narrative practice; it is the bridge between the client's world and the professional's world.

Renowned psychologist Carl Rogers wrote about listening:

> *When I really hear someone, it puts me in touch with him; it enriches my life. It is through hearing people that I have learned all that I know about individuals, about personality, about interpersonal relationships. There is another peculiar satisfaction in really hearing someone: It is like listening to the music of the spheres, because beyond the immediate message of the person, no matter what that might be, there is the universal.*[8]

There are times when we stop listening, or divert the mother's attention to another topic. Why do we do this? Because we think we know what she means? Because we have already decided we know what she will say? Or because she is telling us things we don't want to hear? Do we find ourselves twisting her words slightly to meet our preconceived notion of her problem? Trying to fit her problem into a neat slot that we understand?

Listening with an open mind is a fact of empathy. Empathy is not a skill nor a tool, but rather an "inner experience of sharing in and comprehending the momentary psychological state of another person."[9] Entering into empathy through a desire to connect with and understand another on an emotional level is an experience that can be intrinsically therapeutic for all involved. Miller and Stiver write, "when a person feels another is empathetic, she can often move into action instead of feeling ineffective or immobilized."[10]

We hope that this book will highlight the importance of these skills in understanding and solving breastfeeding problems. This book also represents an essential step in the development of professional lactation consulting services. Without a process such as the Healthy Children

---

[8] Rogers C. *A Way of Being*. Boston: Basic Books; 1980. p. 8.

[9] Schafer R. Generative empathy in the treatment situation. *Psychoanalytic Quarterly*; 28 (3):345; 1959.

[10] Miller JB, Stiver IP. *The Healing Connection: How women form relationships in therapy and in life*. Boston: Beacon Press; 1997.

Eight Level Lactation Consulting Process—the "engineering" component—to structure lactation consultations, helping breastfeeding mothers may sink to the use of "cookie cutter" solutions or maxims, the sign of a technician rather than a professional. When we hear "I always tell my mothers to [fill in your favorite cure here] for sore nipples" we are hearing a cookie cutter or technician-level solution, a maxim. While there are solutions for problems that can be determined to be ineffective or "wrong," there is almost never a single effective or "right" solution that can be applied to every case.[11]

With this book we are hoping to start a conversation about the ways we have come to think about constructing and deconstructing breastfeeding cases. In order to protect client confidentiality, identifying details of these true cases have been altered. These are all cases on which we have consulted. Some of the details contained in this book are blended composites of mothers with whom we have worked during our combined 50-plus years of practice.

We use the convention of the pronoun "we" in referring to the Healthy Children lactation care providers.

Occasionally we have changed the location of the case in order to protect the participants. When other lactation care providers are involved in a case, we refer to them in a generic way without assumptions about background, credentials, knowledge base, or professional training. These case presentations preserve the essential interchanges and details.

In addition to using the Eight Level Process in our consulting work, our practice is directed by the policies and procedures we have agreed upon as a group. Our standard forms, including intake and permission-to-treat forms, assessment tools, and our patient education materials are published by Health Education Associates, Inc.[12]

---

[11] Greenhalgh, T. Narrative based medicine in an evidence based world. *Br Med J*; 318:323–5; 1999.

[12] Health Education Associates, Inc.; 327 Quaker Meeting House Road; East Sandwich, MA 02537; Phone: 508–888–8044; email: info@healthed.cc; web: www.healthed.cc

All consulting sessions include:

1. An intake phase (collection of names and contact information for mother, baby, other family members, and pediatric/obstetric/midwifery/primary health care professionals treating the mother and baby)

2. A consent process (includes a description of what goes on during a consultation, review of and signing of consent form, optional signing of a photo release)

3. The anthropometrics phase (measuring and recording weight and length) prenatal, perinatal, and feeding histories

4. Observation of feeding(s); milk expression; appearance of the mother, her breast, the baby, and milk (if seen); before and after weights may be included, as well as artifacts that may be pertinent

5. Documentation of findings

6. Composing a summary of the plan agreed upon by the mother and the consultant, which includes all referrals to other care providers and support services

7. Giving a copy of the plan to the mother and reiterating follow-up arrangements

8. Writing a summary of the session and communicating with pertinent health care providers

9. Conducting follow-up meetings and/or phone calls, as long as needed, with subsequent documentation and sharing of the plan

We have truncated the assessment process in this book because it is covered in great detail in our previous book on assessment, *Maternal and Infant Assessment for Breastfeeding and Human Lactation: A Guide for the Practitioner*, also published by Jones and Bartlett Publishers. In only the chapter that deals with the importance of assessment do we present an example of assessment. In other chapters we report only pertinent, unusual, or important assessment findings.

We have chosen to share case studies that illustrate common errors made in the problem-solving process of helping mothers with breast-feeding situations. Because of the timing demands of some workplaces, consultants may have learned to use cookie cutter solutions in their work, finding that most women who have X symptom have been found to have Y problem. Like other fields, lactation consulting/counseling has commonly held assumptions about certain symptoms. For example, when a mother describes "sharp stabbing nipple pain," what problem comes to mind? Typically candida overgrowth ("yeast" or "thrush" infection). Yet, there are many other problems that have nipple pain as a symptom, including improper latch, Raynaud's phenomenon, eczema, psoriasis, or neuralgia. We may use a cookie cutter approach to solving breastfeeding problems and be on the right track a good percentage of the time. But what happens when we leap from a symptom to the wrong conclusion without eliciting other pertinent information from history, assessment, and observation? We may cause the mother and baby undue stress, and waste time solving the wrong problem. This may add layers of complexity to solving the actual problem and compensating for the impact of the misdirected intervention.

Providing cookie cutter solutions complicates the problem-solving process, increasing the probability that the consultant may skip over pertinent data that contains clues to the real problem. It takes longer to solve the real problem when one constructs the solution around removing the symptoms without changing the dynamic that is causing the problem. A classic cookie cutter solution is solving nipple soreness by giving the mother a nipple shield without any further assessment to identify the cause of the soreness. The mother may go on to have reduction in her milk supply, the baby may refuse to nurse without the shield, and the mother may continue to have soreness. If the consultant has used cookie cutter thinking to arrive at a solution it is likely that they have not solved the true problem.

The chapters in this book are loosely arranged around the order of the eight levels of the lactation consulting process, with additional chapters illuminating specific consulting issues.

In Chapter 1 we present the Eight Level Lactation Consulting Process, including the rationale for developing such a problem-solving model. We apply the process to six cases with the same symptoms of engorgement but with different histories and assessments. The problem is different in each case. These six cases demonstrate the importance of developing a unique and targeted solution for each consultation. Each level must be addressed; skipping or only partially addressing a level can lead to wrong, incomplete, or inadequate resolution of breastfeeding problems.

In Chapter 2 we explore the importance of history as the first level of the Eight Level Process. The history is elicited through active questioning and listening as well as through documentation, for example, from intake forms and charts.

Chapter 3 examines the use of Level 2: Assess the mother, the baby, and the feeding in the lactation consultation. In this chapter we present cases in which the assessment provides the key to solving the breastfeeding problem. This chapter also includes documentation of the complete assessments of the mothers, the babies, and the feedings included in the chapter.

In Chapter 4 we explore the characteristics of symptoms compared to problems. Symptoms are described by the mother or noted in the baby or the feeding. Problems are formulated by the consultant and explain or underlie the symptoms.

Chapter 5 describes the consulting dilemma of numerators in search of denominators—the situations in which there are multiple, often confusing symptoms, and the one piece of information that anchors these symptoms to a problem may still be missing. These are unusual cases but illustrative of the complexities of lactation consulting.

Chapter 6 presents cases where the mother is stuck. Sometimes a breastfeeding problem revolves around the mother's inability to move along the developmental continuum especially if she, or the baby has experienced a crisis.

In Chapter 7 we explore cases in which the issue is discarding or failing to examine information because it seems uninteresting, unimportant, or irrelevant. The mother or the care provider may believe that a question is not worth asking, or she may have information that has not been considered in the formulation of problems. Cases are provided that serve to illustrate these circumstances.

In Chapter 8 we examine cases where the relationship between psychic pain and breastfeeding presents a problem, including unresolved grief and loss, anxiety about sustaining the infant at the breast and *somatizing*—creating physical pain out of psychic symptoms.

In the cases in Chapter 9 the breastfeeding problems are complicated by family relationships. The issues of siblings, partners, and parents may amplify when a new baby comes into the family and new roles are assumed. With breastfeeding, the intimate relationship between the mother and baby may pose a threat to old family ties.

Chapter 10 explores cases in which the connection between the lactation consultant and the mother, the mother and another mother or mothers, and the mother's connection to her mother provide the key to a rewarding breastfeeding experience.

A glossary is found at the end of the text. Because of the multidisciplinary nature of breastfeeding, definitions of many terms are provided.

Chapter 1

Introduction to the Eight Level Lactation Consulting Process

What I see depends on where I'm at.
—ALBERT EINSTEIN, PHYSICIST (1879–1955)

The Eight Level Lactation Consulting Process emerged from five sources:

1. Our years of clinical practice as lactation consultants
2. Our drive to integrate the multidisciplinary lactation consultant practices at the *Center for Breastfeeding* into a cohesive whole
3. Our supervision of students and clinical interns at the bachelors, masters, and Ph.D. levels
4. The complexity of teaching problem-solving skills to novices and experienced lactation consultants in our Advanced Issues in Lactation Consulting course: Level II Lactation Consulting
5. The insight we have gained by deconstructing cases that have been referred to us by other providers

These five factors didn't come together in a temporal sequence; rather, bits and pieces of insight grew and combined finally emerging into an exciting pattern. When we've shared the Eight Level Lactation Consulting Process with other lactation consultants whose practices we respect they've told us "That's it! That's exactly what I do!" Others have told us that the Eight Level Process has given them insight into where past cases have gone wrong.

1

Our first force toward constructing the Eight Level Lactation Consulting Process is our combined 50-years plus in the clinical practice of lactation consulting. In this book we focus on our practice. Cindy Turner-Maffei had many years of experience in the WIC (the Special Supplemental Nutrition Program for Women, Infants, and Children) program and other public health programs as a nutritionist lactation consultant before joining the Healthy Children faculty. Karin Cadwell is a nurse lactation consultant with experience in the hospital setting, public health agencies, and as a visiting nurse before joining the Healthy Children Project.

The Center for Breastfeeding is a major focus of the Healthy Children Project, providing breastfeeding support services and a telephone warmline to mothers in southeastern Massachusetts, as well as support services to health care workers who are providing care to breastfeeding mothers. Our clinical practice is located at the Center for Breastfeeding.

In the mid-1990s we became interested in the practice of lactation consulting in a new way. When Kajsa Brimdyr, a workplace ethnographer, joined our faculty she challenged us to look at the practice of lactation consulting close-up. We began the job of watching how we do the work of helping women breastfeed. One of the first things that we noted was that although we all agreed to the knowledge base reflected in our policies and procedures manual, each of the lactation consultants at the Center went about the process of consulting in a different way. We began consulting in pairs and were surprised at the questions the other consultant asked. We were amazed at the variety of ways we had come to understand the complex process of consulting. This became our second impetus. We are an interdisciplinary practice so it made sense that we saw the process of consulting through the lens of the disciplines in which we were originally educated. We realized that we needed to develop a consulting process that could be supported by all of the lactation consultants in our practice and among the Healthy Children faculty.

We began to examine models of consultation from other disciplines: nursing models, especially Orem and King, the doctor–patient model, the architect–client model, the purchase of expertise model, and Schein's process consultation model.[1] The process consultation model felt the most comfortable to us, but because it was originally developed for organizational consultants who usually do not have to solve problems quickly, it seemed cumbersome and didn't quite meet the urgency needs we often have as lactation consultants.

---

[1] Schein E. *Process Consultation*. Reading, MA: Addison-Wesley Publishing Company; 1988.

Our third impetus to develop a specific process for lactation consulting came from our supervision of lactation consultant practicums and internships at the bachelors, masters, and Ph.D. levels. Our students were confused by the gap between the practices of lactation consultants they observed in the field and what they were learning in class.

The interns, whether placed with hospital-based lactation consultants, public health lactation consultants, or private practice lactation consultants, tell us the same thing: Many of the lactation care providers they observed do not apply or articulate assessment and critical thinking skills. In addition, each mother does not receive a unique and targeted intervention. The assessment book we wrote with our colleagues Anna Blair and Barbara O'Connor filled an essential need for an assessment text in the field.

We came to understand that much of what they observed was not, in fact, consulting, but technician-level intervention. Their journals reflected that in many of the practices they were observing, almost all the mothers with the same symptoms were treated with the same product, when the product failed to alleviate the symptom another product was applied. Students asked questions such as "What should you do for sore nipples?" They got responses like "For sore nipples use a combination of 1 part cream X, 1 part cream Y, and 1 part cream Z," or "Put a pillow on the mother's lap." These are cookie cutter solutions, appropriate for technicians, but not for professionals. The professional answer is "Find out what problem is causing the nipple soreness, and then plan a directed intervention."

They were concerned that we were teaching them that professional consulting requires unique and targeted solutions for each mother. What our students reported seeing was one-size-fits-all technical solutions.

We recognized that a lactation consulting process would be useful in the classroom as well. We tested and refined the Eight Level Lactation Consulting Process in our Advanced Lactation Consulting course. This five-day class is a unique learning experience.[2] Its focus is the clinical application of theory and technique. The course consists of the didactic consideration of historical and psychosocial models as well as demonstration consultations with mothers who present with complex breastfeeding problems.

This advanced course has been offered all over the United States in settings such as hospitals, WIC programs, physicians' offices, and universities. It has been our privilege to teach both novices and experienced

---

[2] Advanced Issues in Lactation Consulting is the Level II course offered by the Healthy Children Project. Continuing education units (CEUs) for nurses, lactation consultants, childbirth educators, and dietitians are available as well as college credits.

multidisciplinary lactation care providers about critical thinking and problem solving in lactation consulting in this advanced course. You will read about the application of the Eight Level Process in the advanced class in later chapters.

At the Center for Breastfeeding we accept referrals from other care providers. We also see mothers who seek us out after they have been seen by other providers without resolution of their problems. This has have given us insight into what other providers might miss and is the fifth driving force in the development of the process. The Eight Level Lactation Consulting Process includes two levels (Levels 5 and 7) that force the consultant to stop and reconcile the information that has been collected, the problem that has been formulated, and the solutions and interventions that have been planned.

Overview of the Eight Level Lactation Consulting Process

The Eight Level Lactation Consulting Process

- Combines the use of empirical knowledge with critical thinking skills

- Helps to refine choice from a sea of possibilities

- Develops a broader vision of compassionate service to mothers and babies

Each level must be addressed; skipping or only partially addressing a level can lead to wrong, incomplete, or inadequate resolution of breastfeeding problems.

The Eight Level Lactation Consulting Process

1. Level 1: Take a complete *history*.
2. Level 2: *Assess* the mother, the baby, and the feeding.
3. Level 3: Develop a *symptom* list.
4. Level 4: Formulate a *problem* list.
5. Level 5: *Reconcile* the history, assessment, symptoms, and problems.
6. Level 6: Generate and prioritize *solutions* and *plans for interventions*.

Drill Hall Library

Borrowed Items 26/02/2015 16:20
XXXXXXX1373

Item Title	Due Date
6580180426	05/03/2015 23:59
Ethics in clinical practice : an interprofessional approach	
6545444277	05/03/2015 23:59
Facilitating learning in clinical settings	
6580111084	26/03/2015 23:59
Patient _person : interpersonal skills in nursing	
6580019889	26/03/2015 23:59
Caring and communicating : the interpersonal relationship in nursing	
6580199453	26/03/2015 23:59
Person-centred nursing : theory and practice	
6516775511	26/03/2015 23:59
Interpersonal communication in nursing : theory and practice	
6546170006	26/03/2015 23:59
Becoming a reflective practitioner	
6546709770	26/03/2015 23:59
Dignity in healthcare : a practical approach for nurses and midwives	

Overnight loans are due by 9pm on due d
Please retain this receipt for your records

7. Level 7: *Reconcile* prioritized solutions and planned interventions with problems.

8. Level 8: *Evaluate* solutions and interventions.

Applying the Eight Level Lactation Consulting Process

The purpose of applying the Eight Level Process is to ensure that in every case empirical knowledge is combined with critical thinking skills. The first four levels: take a complete history; assess the mother, the baby, and the feeding; develop a symptom list; and formulate a problem list are interactive with each other. If you look at the diagram of the process (Figure 1–1) you can see that we picture these levels as being connected by a series of arrows that go around in a circular motion. That's because the nature of the lactation consulting process is interactive. These four levels rarely are completed in order, one after another. Instead, the lactation consultant must multitask, moving gracefully between each of the first four levels. The activity of assessment of the feeding, for example, shouldn't be forced. If the consultant instructs

FIGURE 1-1 The Eight Level Lactation Consulting Process

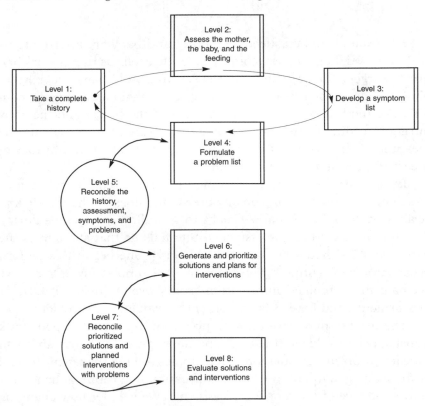

the mother to begin to feed, the pre-feeding interaction of the mother and baby may be missed. If the history is completed first, the baby could be crying and frantic by the time nursing starts.

The consultant must be present in the moment, noting behavior, asking questions, critically thinking, asking "What else do I need to know?" "What is missing from the history, symptoms, and assessment that keeps me from making a problem formulation that unites the findings?" (Figure 1–2).

FIGURE 1–2   The Eight Level Lactation Consulting Process: Interactive Levels 1–4

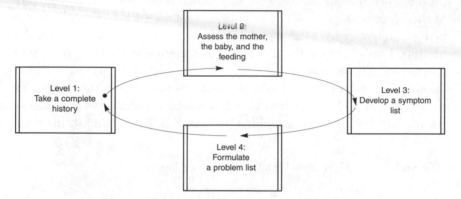

For example, a breastfeeding mother and baby are referred to us with slow weight gain (symptom). The mother tells us that she has had breast surgery (history) and that the seven-day-old baby was born at 37 weeks' gestation (history). However, it is only in assessing the condition of the breast and the performance of the breast and the baby during a feeding (assessment) that we are truly able to evaluate the meaning of the statement the mother has made about her history of breast surgery and the baby's gestation.

By assessing before and after weights, we find that the baby transfers .5 ounces after nursing on one breast and does not have a suck to swallow ratio of lower than 20 sucks to 1 swallow at any time during the 20-minute feeding (assessment). She tells us that she nurses the baby every 3–4 hours by the clock (history). She began this pattern because of her continuing problem of sore nipples (symptom). We evaluate the combined information from Level 1 (history), Level 2 (assessment), and Level 3 (symptoms) to formulate the problem.

The mother may have a low supply of milk as well as poor milk transfer, perhaps due to the supply, perhaps due to the baby's ability to transfer (problem formulation). Her nipples are misshapen at the end of the feeding and have a white compression line running diagonally across the face of the nipple (assessment). We wonder how changing the baby's position for another feeding (assessment) would effect our problem formulation. We observe a second nursing with the baby in a different position and although the mother's nipples are not distorted at the end of the feeding, the suck to swallow ratio remains high, and the baby transfers .3 ounces (assessment). However, the mother reports that she did not experience pain during the second feeding (symptom).

Let's take, for example, a mother who calls on the telephone with the following symptoms.

- Hard breast
- Skin is shiny on the breast
- Breast larger than normal
- Breast warm to the touch
- Breast pain

At the technical level, this list of symptoms would be called "engorgement" and there would be a cookie cutter solution such as pumping, application of cabbage leaves or ice, or soaking the breasts in a basin of warm water—whatever is preferred by the advice giver.

Using the consulting process, in addition to the list of *symptoms* above we would need a *history* and *assessment* before we would be able to determine the *problem*.

Case A:

In collecting the history, we find that the mother is two months postpartum. We also learn that the symptoms appeared for the first time this morning and that her baby slept seven hours without nursing last night for the first time. When we assess her breasts we can see milk leaking from both nipples along with the shiny skin and hardness she described.

What if we had the same list of symptoms in the following scenario?

Case B:

The history indicates that the mother is four days postpartum. The history also indicates that the mother has been nursing only every three to four hours during the daytime, and that the baby spent the first two nights in the hospital nursery at the parents' request. When we assess her breasts there is milk leaking from both nipples.

Or, this scenario?

Case C:

The mother is six days postpartum. According to her history, she has been nursing every hour around the clock since birth. Five years ago she had breast reduction surgery. Assessment of her breasts shows periareolar scarring on both breasts. No milk or leaking is visible. The mother is unable to hand express even a drop of milk from either breast.

Or, this scenario?

Case D:

The mother is 12 days postpartum. According to her history, the baby has consistently refused to nurse on the left breast. Only the left breast has the symptoms.

Or, this scenario?

Case E:

The mother is 10 months postpartum. She tells us that yesterday she left her nursing baby at her sister's house so that she could do back-to-school shopping for her four older children. She was away for six hours. The baby refused to nurse when she picked the baby up at her sister's and has refused to nurse ever since. Assessment shows all of the symptoms in the list. In addition, there is milk leaking from both nipples.

Or, this scenario?

Case F:

The mother is three days postpartum. She has all of the symptoms listed on page 7. She tells us that she had breast augmentation four years ago. She is not planning to breastfeed because she is concerned that the implants could become dislodged.

LEVEL 4   Level 4 of the Eight Level Process is the formulation of a problem based on the history, assessment, and symptoms. As Cases A–F show, the same list of symptoms can have history and assessment that are remarkably different. (Figure 1–3).

FIGURE 1–3   The Eight Level Lactation Consulting Process: Levels 4–8

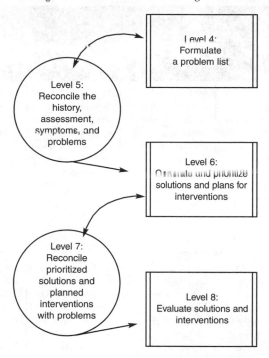

Table 1 illustrates this point. When you look down the list of symptoms (Level 3) you can see that the symptoms are the same in all of the cases. As you read each case, however, you will see that nothing else is constant from one mother to another mother.

When assessed, some mothers have milk leaking readily from the nipple, some do not. This is an important finding as, in the case of a mother who has had surgery, her ducts may not be able to deliver milk, no matter how large her breasts have become.

Also, the history of the mother is an important consideration when combined with the assessment and symptoms. Cases A–F include mothers in the immediate postpartum period who present with the array of symptoms we call engorgement. But determining a plan and intervention for a mother with a 10-month-old who has suddenly stopped nursing (Case E) would not be the same as the plan and intervention for the postpartum mother with implants (Case F) who has no interest in breastfeeding. So, although the symptoms remain the same, the plans are unique and targeted to the specifics of the case.

There are two levels that are shown in Figures 1–1 and 1–3 as circles, Level 5 and Level 7. These are the levels at which we stop and consider what we know and how we know it. This is where we ask ourselves

TABLE 1   Comparison of six case studies with the same symptoms

	Level 1: History	Level 2: Assessment	Level 3: Symptoms	Level 4: Problem Formulation
Case A	The mother is two months postpartum. The symptoms appeared for the first time this morning. The baby slept seven hours without nursing last night for the first time.	Milk is leaking from both nipples along with the shiny skin and hardness mother describes.	Mother describes hard breast with shiny skin; breast larger than normal and warm to the touch; breast pain.	Milk production is not in balance with change in feeding pattern.
Case B	The mother is four days postpartum. The mother has been nursing only every three to four hours during the daytime, and the baby spent the first two nights in the hospital nursery at the parents' request.	There is milk leaking from both nipples. The physical symptoms the mother describes are present.	Mother describes hard breast with shiny skin; breast larger than normal and warm to the touch; breast pain.	Inadequate feeding frequency with the potential of inadequate ongoing milk production. Temporary over-fullness of breast.
Case C	The mother is six days postpartum. She has been nursing every hour around the clock since birth. Five years ago she had breast reduction surgery.	Periareolar scarring is visible on both breasts. No milk or leaking is visible. The mother is unable to hand express even one drop of milk from either breast.	Mother describes hard breast with shiny skin; breast larger than normal and warm to the touch; breast pain.	Potential inability to deliver milk due to non-patent ducts.

TABLE 1   Comparison of six case studies with the same symptoms (continued)

	Level 5: Reconcile the H, A, S, & P	Level 6: Generate & Prioritize Solutions & Plans for Intervention	Level 7: Reconcile Solutions & Interventions with Problems	Level 8: Evaluate Solutions & Interventions
Case A	The history, assessment, symptoms, and problem reconcile.	Hand express, pump, or use a water bath depending on whether the mother wants to collect the milk to use later. Keep breasts as soft and comfortable as possible.	Because the problem is temporary (the baby may not sleep through the night tonight) the mother may have to repeat this process. The problem and solutions do reconcile.	The mother and baby will be able to balance the milk supply as the baby's needs and developmental stages change.
Case B	The history, assessment, symptoms, and problem reconcile. More assessment is needed of baby's condition and of feeding.	Teach parents about expected breastfeeding pattern. Ensure pediatric follow-up and weight checks for baby. Ensure adequate intake of baby. Teach mother to pump or hand express. Feed collected milk to baby if needed.	The problem and solutions do reconcile.	The baby must be fed 10–12 times a day including night feedings. The baby should make an adequate weight gain by pediatric standards.
Case C	The history, assessment, symptoms, and problem reconcile.	Determine an alternate source of nutrition and feeding method for the baby if needed. Evaluate milk transfer. Try pumping or hand expression. Institute comfort techniques and a more appropriate feeding pattern.	The problem and solutions do reconcile.	Mother will enjoy feeding her baby. Baby will be adequately nourished according to pediatric standards.

continues

TABLE 1   Comparison of six case studies with the same symptoms (continued)

	Level 1: History	Level 2: Assessment	Level 3: Symptoms	Level 4: Problem Formulation
Case D	The mother is 12 days postpartum. The baby has consistently refused to nurse on the left breast. Only the left breast has the symptoms.	The left breast is 50% larger than the right. The baby refuses the breast in every position attempted. Milk can be expressed. Left axilla area is also enlarged with painful nodes palpated.	Mother describes hard breast with shiny skin; breast larger than normal and warm to the touch; breast pain.	Possible breast disease.[1,2] Possible pediatric problem such as tortocollis or birth trauma.
Case E	The mother is 10 months postpartum. Yesterday she left her nursing baby at her sister's house so that she could do back-to-school shopping for her 4 older children. She was away for 6 hours. The baby refused to nurse when she picked the baby up at her sister's and has refused to nurse ever since.	Assessment shows all of the symptoms that the mother described. In addition, there is milk leaking from both nipples.	Mother describes hard breast with shiny skin; breast larger than normal and warm to the touch; breast pain.	Nursing strike
Case F	The mother is three days postpartum. She tells us that she had breast augmentation four years ago. She is not planning to breastfeed because she is concerned that the implants would be dislodged.	All of the symptoms described by the mother are observed. In addition three-inch scars are present on the chest wall under both breasts.	Mother describes hard breast with shiny skin; breast larger than normal and warm to the touch; breast pain.	Physiologic process of Lactogenesis is the same in mothers who want to breastfeed as those who don't choose to breastfeed.

[1]Goldsmith HS. Milk-rejection sign of cancer. AM J. Surg. 1974, 127 (3): 280.
[2]Saber A. Dardik, Ibrahim I.M., Wolodiger F. The Milk Rejection Sign: A Natural Tumor Marker. AM Surg 1996, 62 (12): 998.

TABLE 1 Comparison of six case studies with the same symptoms (continued)

	Level 5: Reconcile the H, A, S, & P	Level 6: Generate & Prioritize Solutions & Plans for Intervention	Level 7: Reconcile Solutions & Interventions with Problems	Level 8: Evaluate Solutions & Interventions
Case D	The history, assessment, symptoms, and problem reconcile.	Refer mother to physician for breast evaluation. Institute pumping, hand expression. Institute comfort techniques. Refer baby to pediatrician.	The problem and solutions do reconcile.	Mother should have ongoing breast evaluation. Breast cancer may be diagnosed up to five years after this behavior in the baby.
Case E	The history, assessment, symptoms, and problem reconcile.	Hand express or pump for comfort. Do not force baby to the breast, rather, try nursing when baby is asleep or sleepy. Bring baby to visit with another breastfeeding couple.	The solutions and problems do reconcile.	Nursing will resume as before. Mother will have an increased awareness of potential of hurting the baby's feelings. Nursing strikes are one of the ways baby's can demonstrate unhappiness.
Case F	The history, assessment, symptoms, and problem reconcile.	Help the mother achieve maximum comfort during involution. Try compression to accelerate involution and decrease pain.	The solutions and problems do reconcile.	The mother involutes with minimum discomfort.

"Does what I'm thinking make sense?" These two levels are essential to ensuring the highest level of care for the mothers and babies we serve. At Level 5, we stop and reconcile the history, assessment, symptoms, and the problem we have formulated. In order to move on to generate and prioritize solutions and plans for interventions (Level 6) we must be sure that the problems we have formulated reconcile with the history, assessment, and symptoms. Ask yourself, are there other assessments that should be made that are outside of my scope of practice and require a referral to another provider for more information? Diagnostic tests? If I had more time, would my assessment be different?

The Center for Breastfeeding is set up like a living room. It is a comfortable area that allows us to assess breastfeedings in a variety of positions and using a variety of furniture. This is helpful since the mother can nurse in the way that is most like the way she would nurse at home. Although we do have private areas to consult with one mother and baby at a time, our usual practice is to accommodate as many mothers and babies that come at one time. The mothers like to talk with each other and this takes time pressure off of us to finish up with one dyad, and get them out the door before the next appointment. We may have a mother and baby who stay for several hours. We can assess multiple feedings, the mother's attention to feeding cues, and try a variety of positions and techniques. We encourage you to ask yourself at Level 5, "If I had more time, would I assess something different?" and "How have the constraints of time effected my practice?"

Like Level 5, Level 7 is one where we stop and reconcile our thinking. Do the solutions we've planned integrate appropriately with the problem we've formulated? We ask ourselves if our solutions are evidenced-based. We ask if the solutions have been shown to be effective for each of the problems we have formulated. Do any of the solutions contradict each other? Will any solution or intervention cause harm? Use up-to-date breastfeeding texts and research articles to guide your selection of targeted solutions and interventions. Be sure to read any information thoroughly. Ask yourself if there are any exceptions to the intervention or solution. Look up words in the index and glossary in the back of the book to see if there is additional information in another section of the book that might make a difference for this mother and baby.

Ask yourself whether the plans and solutions you have prioritized are within your scope of practice to recommend. Is a referral to another practitioner needed? Have you compromised the outcome for the mother and baby by not working with other members of the health care team? An example of this is the recommendation of a home remedy, when a prescription may result in a better outcome.

Levels 5 and 7 are also the two levels at which we are mandated to stop and check with the mother and baby about what we are thinking. We tell the mother what we think the problems are and why they make sense to us based on the history, assessment, and symptoms. Do they make sense to her? We have had the experience of the mother telling us that we have misunderstood her symptom or history, she doesn't feel comfortable about our problem formulation, or she would like us to assess something else. Again at Level 7, we discuss the way we are thinking with the mother. This is the level where we find out that she doesn't want to nurse more often, pump, or use an at-breast feeding system. She tells us that she's confused, it seems like too much work, she doesn't feel confident, or doesn't have transportation. It is also the level at which she can agree with our plan. Level 7, like Level 5, if skipped or rushed can have disastrous results not only because of the "buy-in" from the mother, but because of the critical thinking that is part of each of these two levels.

Further Reading

Brimdyr K. "Lactation Management: A community of practice" in *Reclaiming Breastfeeding in the United States: Promotion, Protection and Support.* K. Cadwell, ed. Sudbury, MA: Jones and Bartlett Publishers; 2003.

Cadwell K, Turner-Maffei C, O'Connor B, Blair A. *Maternal and Infant Assessment for Breastfeeding and Human Lactation: A Guide for the Practitioner.* Sudbury, MA: Jones and Bartlett Publishers; 2002.

Schein E. *Process Consultation.* Reading, MA: Addison-Wesley Publishing Company; 1988.

Weiss A. *Process Consulting.* San Francisco: Jossey-Bass/Pfeiffer; 2002.

Discussion Questions

1. What restraints have you experienced that keep you from using all of the levels in the Eight Level Process with each consultation? How can you modify your work environment so that every mother and baby receives a professional consultation rather than a technical, cookie cutter solution?

2. Which of the levels are the most natural for you? Which do you think are the most difficult? Why?

3. The lactation consultants at the Center for Breastfeeding found that working in pairs was enlightening. Is this something that you can do? How would you go about arranging such a collaboration?

Chapter 2

History

"Discovery consists of seeing what everybody has seen and thinking what nobody has thought."

—ALBERT VON SZENT-GYORGYI, BIOCHEMIST
(1893–1986)

This chapter addresses the crucial history-taking phase of consultation. In order to fully understand the problem the mother and baby are experiencing careful listening, questioning, and thinking are needed.

Ashley & Jared

We met Ashley and Jared while teaching the Lactation Consulting Level II course. During this class, we interview women with difficult breastfeeding problems. In the tradition of this course, the participants, the mother, and her family members sit in a circle of chairs. Each workshop participant asks one question of the mom. Then the next participant asks one question, and so forth until everyone has had an opportunity to pose a question. The goal of this exercise is to listen actively to the mother and her family, to examine one's own thinking process (and that of others), and to craft one's question wisely to gather information and clues to the nature of the problem.

Kristin, who worked for the hosting hospital, had recruited Ashley to present her experience to the class. Kristin told us that she had been working with Ashley for some time. Ashley had been coming to the hospital-sponsored breastfeeding clinic more than once weekly for help with nursing her baby.

> *Ashley entered the room. She looked a bit frazzled. She was laden with a diaper bag, a large drink container, and an oversized purse, while pushing a jogging stroller containing a sleepy Jared. She sat down with a sigh in the chair Kristin had found for her, and gratefully accepted the offer of some tea and a snack. When she was settled, we explained that we were a group of experienced breastfeeding care providers who were interested in learning about her experience and in watching ourselves go about the process of questioning. We told her that we were trying to understand how to best help women solve breastfeeding problems. She said that she was happy to help, and so we began to ask one question each.*

Participant 1: *"Hi Ashley. Thanks for coming to meet with us today. Can you tell us how old your baby is, and what concerns bring you here today?"*

Ashley: *"Jared is ten weeks old today. Well, breastfeeding has been tougher than I thought it would be. Right now, Jared's weight gain hasn't been so good, so I'm hoping to get some more tips."*

Participant 2: *"Can you tell us how much he weighed at birth and how he much he weighs right now?"*

Ashley: *"He weighed 5 pounds, 11 ounces at birth. Now he weighs almost 9 pounds. For a while, he was gaining better, but lately he's slowed down."*

Participant 2: *"Was he born prematurely?"*

Ashley: *"About a week early. The doctor said he was full-term, but just a peanut."*

Kristin: *"I have his growth chart here if anyone would like to take a look."*

A crowd formed around her chair.

Participant 3: *"Can you tell us what you've done to try to help with this situation?"*

Ashley: *"Lots of things: pumping, feeding him pumped milk, increasing my fluids, even some formula. Nothing seems to help. I'm about worn out."*

Participant 4: *"Tell us about that 'worn out' feeling, please."*

Ashley: *"I've had diarrhea for the last several days. I might be fighting the flu, or something. Usually I can stop diarrhea by just eating a few grains of rice, but this time that hasn't worked. Otherwise, I'm just really tired. I'm not sleeping very well, I have no appetite, and I can't even get up the energy to walk with the baby. My house will probably never be clean again. But, that's OK, he's the most important thing. I just want to give him the very best I can."*

Participant 5: *"I commend you on your commitment to your baby, Ashley. How was the pregnancy and birth?"*

Ashley: *"It's a little embarrassing. I didn't even know I was pregnant until about the sixth month. I started having some pains in my stomach, and my doctor told me I was pregnant. Oh, I was so happy! I gave that doctor a big kiss! We've been married for eleven years now. We tried to conceive for years, but didn't have any luck. Finally, we just came to peace with that, and focused on our four-footed children (you know, our pets). The pregnancy was pretty healthy, a little trouble with my blood pressure, but OK. The labor was long, and ended up in a cesarean section. But Jared*

was amazing; he took my breast right
on the delivery table. My husband
was so proud of him—a breast man
from the start, he said!"

Participant 6:   "And how did breastfeeding go in the
early days?"

Ashley: "OK. I had some soreness, a couple of
breast infections, and thrush. Kristin
and the other women here were wonderful. They've helped me so much. I
don't know how I would have gotten
through all of this without them."

Thoughts

Our thoughts: Two episodes of mastitis and a case of thrush are a lot
for the first ten weeks. Is there some mechanical problem causing the
breast inflammation? Could her immune system be suppressed? Is
she anemic? Could she have other endocrine problems (history of
infertility)?

Participant 7:   "How long ago was the last infection?
Have all of the thrush symptoms gone
away?"

Ashley: "Oh, all those things ended at least
two weeks ago, I'd say. I wish I could
just feel stronger, I seem to catch everything that's going around. Thank God
Jared's been healthy. I guess my milk is
helping him."

Participant 8:   "I have no doubt that your milk is
helping him. Take us through an aver-
age day, would you? Tell us about
feeding, sleeping, diaper changes, etc."

Ashley then recounted the prior day, noting at least
10 breastfeedings, 2 dirty diapers and numerous wet
ones, 3 naps for the baby, a 5-hour stretch of sleep during the night, and 5 hours of fussy, inconsolable
behavior.

Participant 9:   "How typical would you say yesterday
was?"

Ashley:	*"It was typical of Jared in the last 10 days or so. Before that he was not so sleepy and fussy."*
Participant 10:	*"You mentioned some trouble with your blood pressure in pregnancy. Are you taking any medication?"*
Ashley:	*"No. My blood pressure was fine after delivery. I don't believe in taking anything unless it's absolutely necessary. I got through both my breast infections without any medication. I don't want to do anything that would hurt my baby."*
Participant 11:	*"Has anything changed in the last two weeks? Have you eaten any new foods, changed anything else about your life or Jared's?"*
Ashley:	*"Let me think . . . I'm still taking some acidophilus. I'm hoping to avoid future problems with yeast. The pediatrician suggested taking it, and said it wouldn't hurt Jared. I've been so tired in the last week that I haven't gone out for my daily walk. Nothing else has changed that I can think of."*
Participant 12:	*"What does the pediatrician have to say about Jared's growth?"*
Ashley:	*"Well, he says he's not worried, that lots of big women like me have little tiny babies. I've called a couple of times this week, but the nurse says it's normal for babies to be fussy around this age."*
Participant 13:	*"Can you tell us about Jared's bowel movements?"*
Ashley:	*"Well, those are different lately, come to think of it. His poop is sort of drier and smaller in quantity than it used to be, a little darker in color, too."*

Participant 14: *"You may want to mention that to your pediatrician. What other behavior of Jared's troubles you?"*

Ashley: *"His fussiness and his sleepiness I guess. It seems funny to complain about a baby sleeping too much, but it's like he's always exhausted. He goes to sleep cranky and wakes up cranky. He doesn't enjoy the games his dad plays with him, like airplane, that he used to love. He frowns a lot and looks worried."*

True to reported form, Jared began to stir in his stroller, fussing and scowling as he opened his eyes to find himself the center of attention. Ashley scooped him up, talking soothingly, and determined that he had a wet diaper. As she changed him, she asked if we'd like to see the diaper. It was a soaking wet cloth diaper with a slim green-brown streak of fecal matter in its center. Ashley reported that this was a smaller amount of stool than he normally produced at this time of day. We placed him on the infant scale and recorded his pre-feeding weight. Ashley asked Kristin to hold Jared for a minute, and excused herself to go to the ladies room. She returned a few minutes later, apologizing for leaving, and telling us that she was feeling wiped out from the diarrhea.

Participant 15: *"Could you tell us more about the diarrhea? Have you made any trips out of the country lately? Eaten any undercooked meat? Have your pets been ill?"*

Ashley: *"No trips out of the country. No, I don't eat much meat at all. I don't digest it well. And no, the pets haven't been ill—they certainly haven't had as much attention as they'd like, but they're healthy. I have a tendency toward diarrhea, but I must have the flu now, or another bug, because I can't control it."*

Participant 16: *"Do you have food allergies?"*

Ashley:	*"No, there are just some foods that give me instant diarrhea. Kristin and I have wondered if it is something I'm eating that's upsetting Jared. I hardly ever eat dairy, but we tried changing some other things. So far, it hasn't helped."*

As Ashley spoke, she prepared to breastfeed Jared. He calmed down when she cradled him to the breast, opened his mouth, and slurped onto the breast. "Ouch," Ashley said, "you must be hungry—that wasn't a great latch." As she spoke, he pulled back his head slightly, and relaxed his jaw, opening to about a 140° angle and almost immediately entering into a 2:1 or 1:1 suck to swallow pattern. After asking permission to observe quietly, participants filed behind the nursing couple, observing the feeding position, latch, and behavior. A few made small suggestions for ways to optimize the feeding, which Ashley immediately implemented. When the suck/swallow ratio increased, she instinctively began alternate massage, which quickly brought the ratio back into a nutritive pattern.

Participant 17:	*"Sounds like he's getting a good intake of milk. Earlier you mentioned that you had tried pumping and feeding extra milk to Jared. Could you tell us how that went?"*
Ashley:	*"It took me a while to get used to the pump that the clinic loaned to me. At first I was pumping less than ½ ounce, but in a few days I could get more than 3 ounces in about 10 minutes. I fed him a lot of that milk by cup, but he usually didn't take it, or spit it up afterward. My husband had some luck getting him to take it, but I noticed that when we fed him the pumped milk he didn't feed as much at the next feeding."*
Participant 18:	*"You mentioned that you were not able to become pregnant for years.*

	Can you tell us more about that? Did you go to a fertility specialist, and if so what did you learn? Oh, and do you have any history of endocrine problems, like thyroid disease or menstrual problems?"
Ashley:	*"Whoa. That was more than one question! Yes, my husband and I tried for years to get pregnant. He got worked up: no problems. I got worked up; no problems except they thought my weight might be a problem. I've always been a really large woman."*
Participant 18:	*"Pardon me for disagreeing, but you don't seem like a 'really large woman' to me."*
Ashley:	*"Oh, that's because I had gastric bypass surgery a couple of years ago, and lost about 150 pounds. I still think of myself as big. My doctor said that it's probably the weight loss that made me fertile. I gained about 50 pounds back with the pregnancy."*
Participant 19:	*"Have you had a problem with diarrhea since the surgery?"*
Ashley:	*"At first, yes. But then I learned that eating literally a tablespoon of rice would stop me right up. Until lately."*
Participant 20:	*"What has been happening with your weight lately? Have you been losing, maintaining, or gaining?*
Ashley:	*"I think I was down about 20 pounds from delivery at my 6 week checkup. After that, I don't know. I'd say I've lost some more weight. I almost fit in my regular clothes."*

At this point, all the participants had asked a question (some had cleverly managed to fit three or four questions into one sentence). While Ashley burped Jared, and moved him to the other breast, the group huddled to review findings.

Level 1—History

Significant history for mother includes infertility, gastric bypass surgery, late prenatal care, cesarean birth, two bouts of mastitis, a *Candida* infection of the breast, and ongoing problems with diarrhea.

The baby's history includes fussy and sleepy behavior in the last two weeks, and weight gain problems.

Level 2—Assessment

Mother and baby seem adept at feeding. Minor changes were made to optimize positioning. Mother denies any pain on feeding. Milk flow is observed from both breasts between feeding, and reported pumped volumes are within expected range. [Later post-feeding weight showed a combined transfer of 3.9 ounces from both breasts.]

Level 3—Symptoms

- Mother: exhaustion, diarrhea, concern about baby
- Baby: fussiness, sleepiness, scant bowel movements

Level 4—Problem Formulation

- Gastrointestinal problem with baby and/or mother (parasite, celiac disease, allergy, etc.)
- Child small for age

Level 5—Reconcile the History, Assessment, Symptoms, and Problems

As we discussed this step, one of us asked Ashley one more question:

> *"You mentioned that you didn't want to take anything that might harm the baby. I know that you must have some vitamins you need to take after the gastric bypass surgery. Are you still taking them?"*

Ashley: *"No. I stopped when I found out I was pregnant. I took the prenatal vitamins during pregnancy, but nothing since."*

A flurry of comments came from the participants. Two began talking about intrinsic factor, the chemical released in the stomach that assists in the body's production of B12. Others ran to consult with the texts at the front of the room. Ashley and Jared sat quietly nursing, suddenly the calm eye in the center of a storm of chatter and activity.

Ashley:	*"What? What did I say? Is it bad that I'm not taking the vitamins?"*
Kristin:	*"It raises an interesting possibility for what's going on both with you and with Jared: a vitamin deficiency."*
Ashley:	*"Wow. After the bypass, they did tell me that I should always take that vitamin, but I just thought the prenatal one would be better. Frankly my OB told me I didn't need to take the prenatal vitamins any longer, I haven't even thought about my bypass vitamins."*

This finding caused us to add another potential problem to the list: pernicious anemia in mother and/or baby. Pernicious anemia results from inadequate vitamin B12 absorption due to inadequate production and secretion of intrinsic factor.[1]

- Vitamin B12 deficiency in mother and/or child[2]

Level 6—Generate and Prioritize Solutions and Plans for Interventions

- Immediate pediatric visit for Jared to assess growth and vitamin needs (Jared's doctor has an office in the hospital building where we are meeting. Kristin immediately secured an appointment for that afternoon.)

- Immediate appointment with Ashley's internist to discuss B12 needs, as well as other nutrients

- Continued breastfeeding support and follow-up

---

[1] Mahan LK, Escott-Stump S. *Krause's Food, Nutrition & Diet Therapy, 10th ed.* Philadelphia: W. B. Saunders; 2000, pp. 95–97.

[2] Grange DK, Finlay JL. Nutritional vitamin B12 deficiency in a breastfed infant following maternal gastric bypass. *Pediatr Hematol Oncol* 11(3):311–8; 1994.

Martens WS, Martin LF, Berlin CM. Failure of a nursing infant to thrive after the mother's gastric bypass for morbid obesity. *Pediatrics* 86(5):777–8; 1990.

CDC. Neurologic Impairment in Children Associated with Maternal Dietary Deficiency of Cobalamin—Georgia, 2001. *MMWR Morbi Mortal Wkly Rep.* 52(4):61–4; 2003.

Level 7—Reconcile Prioritized Solutions and Planned Interventions with Problems

This plan seems to account for the currently known problems. Additional planning may be needed after the physician visits.

Level 8—Evaluate Solutions and Interventions

Because we met with Ashley on the first day of a five-day course, we were able to learn more about her case throughout the week. Kristin reported the next day that Jared's doctor thought he might be B12 deficient, and prescribed an over-the-counter infant vitamin to provide for this need. Ashley got in to see her doctor later that day and received a B12 shot.

Later in the week, Ashley dropped in to visit the class when she came for breastfeeding clinic again on Friday. She looked rested and much calmer.

> *"I'm a different woman. I feel like I've slept for the first time in months. My diarrhea has nearly gone away. Jared seems a little happier, too. I can't thank you all enough for helping me. I feel stupid about forgetting to take the vitamin."*
>
> *The participants reassured her that mothering is a bizarre and wonderful journey, and thanked her for such a powerful lesson on the importance of thinking about the big picture.*

Maria & Isabel

We were teaching the Lactation Consulting Level II course again at a hospital in the western United States, when we met Maria and her little girl, Isabel. One of the class participants, Lourdes, invited Maria, a client she met in her work as a public health nutritionist, to be interviewed by the class. Maria agreed to present her situation.

> *Lourdes greeted Maria and helped her to find a comfortable seat. Lourdes set up some toys on the rug for Isabel. Maria put the baby down on the rug, but she immediately protested, holding up her arms to her mom. Maria scooped her up with a sigh, and placed the baby on her lap, facing out. Isabel kept her head tucked down, and clung to her mom, but her eyes darted around the room, looking furtively about, her brow furrowed, and her*

mouth turned down. Maria seemed a bit nervous to find herself the focus of 20 strangers, but smiled shyly. We explained to Maria how the class would like to explore her situation, and told her that she was free to move about, to feed Isabel at will, to pass on any questions she didn't want to answer, etc.

Participant 1:   *"Maria, thank you for coming to be with us today, and for bringing your adorable baby. Would you tell us how breastfeeding has been going?"*

Maria took a deep breath.

Maria: *"I'm worried about Isabel. She doesn't seem to be growing well. She is fussy; I just can't put her down. I think breastfeeding is good for most babies, but I'm not sure if it's good for her."*

Participant 2:   *"Is Isabel your first child?"*

Maria: *"No. My husband and I have seven children between us, four of mine, two of his, and Isabel, our first baby together."*

Participant 3:   *"Did you nurse any of your other children? How old are your kids?"*

Maria: *"Yes, I nursed all four of mine plus Isabel. Our other kids are 16, 14, 12, 11, 8, and 5."*

Participant 4:   *"Wow! You certainly have your hands full! How old is Isabel now and how much does she weigh?"*

Maria: *"She just had her six-month checkup last week, and she weighed 14 pounds."*

Participant 5:   *"How much did she weigh at birth?"*

Maria: *"6 pounds, eight ounces."*

Participant 6:   *"I'd like to ask Lourdes and Maria if either one has a copy of Isabel's growth chart."*

Lourdes: *"Yes, I brought a copy."*

At this point, the questioning stopped briefly as the class moved over to Lourdes' chair to examine the copy of Isabel's growth chart. The chart indicated that Isabel had skimmed along the twenty-fifth percentile for weight during the first two months, then fallen to the fifth percentile, where she continued to hover. Her length for age had held steady at the twenty-fifth percentile since birth, putting her current weight-to-length ratio between the tenth and twenty-fifth percentile. Her head circumference began at the seventy-fifth percentile, dropped to the fiftieth at the four-month mark, the last time it was noted.

Participant 7:	*"What does Isabel's pediatrician have to say about her growth?"*
Maria:	*"Well, we've seen a different nurse or doctor every time we've been to the clinic. At the last visit, the doctor didn't seem too concerned. She said my milk might not be rich enough, and that I should start giving the baby carrots, that that would help her grow. I tried giving her carrots every meal for the next two days, but she just spat them up, or turned her head away."*

Isabel's behavior caught our eye. She appeared to be struggling to hold onto eye contact with her mother, struggling to ignore the many admiring participants in the room who tried to interest her in conversing with them by making faces and little sounds. Because her mother held her facing out toward the group, she had twisted her head as far as it could go to track her mother. Her little hands were clenched tightly to her mother's shirt. We wondered if she was suffering from stranger and/or separation anxiety.

Participant 8:	*"Is she eating or drinking anything besides your milk now?"*
Maria:	*"Some baby cereal and fruit. I haven't fed her anything else. My husband and kids try to give her tastes of things they're eating. She will eat a little bit, sometimes."*
Participant 9:	*"What worries you most about Isabel?"*
Maria:	*"Different things every day. Maybe she has a stomach problem. Maybe she's spoiled. I don't know. I tried to get the*

doctor to refer her to a stomach specialist, but she said she wanted to just
watch the baby and see how she did
with the carrots. As if she'll be the doctor we'll see next time."

Participant 10:   *"Can you tell us about her diapers?
How often does she poop and pee?
What does her poop look like?"*

Maria: *"She poops about once a day. It's usually just a small stain of runny, yel-
low-green poop. She pees all the
time—no problems there."*

Participant 11:   *"Can you tell us more about what
makes you think she has a stomach
problem? Any other symptoms?"*

Maria: *"She just seems like she's in pain. Look
at her face right now, see her frowning?
That's what she's like. I can't get anything done around the house. I have a
large family to cook, clean, and wash
for. My husband works two jobs to
support us all. The kids help out some,
but there's a lot to do. Sometimes I can
put the baby down on the floor and she
starts to play with her toys, but if I
move away, she starts to cry. She can't
be alone for one second. When the kids
are home from school, they can keep
her happy for a few minutes, but if I go
out of her sight, she starts to cry. I feel
like I should sit down and rock her
when she looks like that. I can't get anything done!"*

Participant 12:   *"This sounds very stressful, Maria.
How are you doing with that?"*

Maria: *"Not so good. I'm tense all the time. My
husband says that nursing is the prob-
lem. His ex didn't nurse their kids, and
he says they were a lot happier. He used
to like that I nursed Isabel, but now
he's pushing me to stop."*

Participant 13:	*"And what about you, Maria? How do you feel about that?"*
Maria:	*"I nursed all my kids for the first year. How could I not do the same for her? It's one of the only things that makes her happy. How can I stop? I just want to make sure it's not hurting her."*

As if to demonstrate her point, Isabel began to push up her mom's shirt. After asking if it was OK to nurse her, Maria turned the baby around toward her, dropped her bra cup. Her breasts appeared full and round. Her nipples were flat in appearance. Isabel latched on. Her mouth position was rather narrow, and the phase of non-nutritive (high suck to swallow ratio) lasted for the first two minutes or so. A pattern of 2:1 and 1:1 sucking then began. Isabel was startled by the loud noise of a book hitting the floor and detached from the breast. We were able to observe that Maria's flat nipple had everted inside Isabel's mouth, and her milk ejection reflex was working, as three or more sprays of milk hit Isabel's cheek, tempting her to latch back on.

We had been thinking the symptom of low weight gain might correlate with inadequate stimulation due to flat or inverted nipples, but the sight of the everted nipple indicates that nipple stimulation is causing a neurohormonal response.

Participant 14:	*"Do you have any breast or nipple discomfort?"*
Maria:	*"Does it hurt when she nurses? Not usually. Sometimes she pinches me with her fingers."*
Participant 15:	*"How often does she nurse?"*
Maria:	*"About every three hours."*
Participant 16:	*"Throughout the day and night? So, eight feedings a day or so?"*
Maria:	*"Yes, I guess so. Sometimes she nurses more in the night than she does in the day. She sleeps right next to our bed, and sometimes I wake up to find her nursing. I must have moved her into our bed in my sleep."*

This participant then asked Maria to give a detailed accounting of the past 24 hours. After Maria recounted the day's feedings and activities, the group noted that Isabel had completed seven breastfeedings, plus about two tablespoons of infant cereal in the morning, and three tablespoons of applesauce in the evening. When asked if this was a typical day, Maria agreed.

Participant 17:   *"Do you or your children have any food allergies?"*

Maria: *"I can't drink milk—it gives me a stomachache and the runs. My kids are totally healthy. No problems."*

Participant 18:   *"Any history of respiratory or skin allergies in your family?"*

Maria: *"No. My husband has some troubles with the pollen sometimes, and I have some skin rashes from cleaning products, but the kids are OK."*

Isabel ended the feeding at this point. Maria patted her back absently, checked her diaper, and placed her on the floor. Isabel picked up a toy, then looked around at all the strangers in the room, and began to cry. After a few minutes, Maria picked her up, and sat her back on her lap, where Isabel resumed her focus on trying to make eye contact with mom.

Participant 19:   *"It sounds like your life is incredibly busy, Maria. How are you holding up?"*

Maria: *"I'm tired all the time. It's hard to get out of bed in the morning. I have six kids to feed and get off to school. Then there's the baby who needs to be to fed, bathed, and dressed. And the laundry, the shopping, you know, it never ends. And my mother—she lives in Mexico—she's been really sick. I've been driving back and forth to see her every month."*

Lourdes was the last participant to ask a question. Before she did so, she quickly jotted a note, and handed it to Maria, who read it and nodded to Lourdes.

Lourdes:	*"Thanks for giving me permission to bring this up, Maria. I just remembered that you were taking some medication for depression during this pregnancy. Are you still taking that medication and how are you feeling emotionally?"*
Maria:	*"I stopped taking the pills during pregnancy. We couldn't afford the prescription. I'm still feeling pretty depressed, actually."*
Lourdes:	*"Have you told your doctor about this? I'm sure they could help you. We can find a way to get your prescription paid for."*
Maria:	*"I don't think the doctor can help me, I'm taking care of this myself, getting myself back together. And if you're talking about Medicaid, don't get me started. I don't do that. I pay for what I need, that's my way."*
Faculty 1:	*"I hear you on that Maria. Have you experienced depression at other times in your life?"*
Maria:	*"I never got depressed until I broke up with my ex. A friend of mine told me I needed help, so I got some counseling, and took some medicine for about six months. Then I got off the drug, and got my life back together. I was OK until this last year. I got really moody almost as soon as I got pregnant with Isabel. I hadn't planned to get pregnant, but my husband and I were happy about it."*
Faculty 2:	*"How was the pregnancy and birth for you physically?"*
Maria:	*"Other than the depression, it was OK. My blood is low, so I had to take a lot of iron, which doesn't sit too*

> well with me. The birth was fast—
> from first pain to delivery it was
> about three hours. I was out of the
> hospital and back home in less than a
> day. I felt great at first. The older kids
> and my husband were really sweet
> and my mother came up and took
> care of us for a while. That was a
> good time."

At this point, each participant had asked a question. We asked Maria if she would prefer to listen to us talk through our impressions, or to leave the room and return when we were done. She opted to stay in the room with us, which we have found generally the most helpful and transparent option, as it allows us all to explore what we're thinking and get more information and clarification at the same time.

 ## Level 1—History

- Maria: Grand multipara, experienced breastfeeder, history of depression and anemia

- Isabel: W/A fifth percentile, slow weight gain

 ## Level 2—Assessment

Maria's nipples appear flat, but are seen to evert on suckling. Evidence of milk flow is seen. Baby shows ability to elicit milk flow. Baby looks worried or in pain.

 ## Level 3—Symptoms

- Maria: Concern about baby, relatively flat affect, and recurrent depression
- Isabel: Slow weight gain, apparent anxiety, reported irritability, scanty bowel movements

 ## Level 4—Problem Formulation

Participants formulated the following possible problems:

- Inadequate milk production relative to inadequate drainage
- Inadequate milk intake

- Attachment difficulties

- Gastrointestinal problem in baby, or possible allergy to some substance consumed by mother or baby

- Probable untreated depression, perhaps resulting in difficulty responding to feeding cues

- Possible anemia, possibly resulting in impaired problem solving

🏅 Level 5—Reconcile the History, Assessment, Symptoms, and Problems

> *As the participants mulled over these theories, one participant, Tina, moved over to Maria's chair and had a whispered conversation with her. We noticed Maria shaking her head, and talking. Tina then came back to the group and said, "Maria wants us to know that she started taking an antidepressant again four months ago. She is buying it when she goes to Mexico, and bringing it back. "Aah," we all replied. [Tina, a nurse who has family in Mexico herself, later shared with us that the fact that Maria traveled monthly to Mexico to see her mother made her think of the possibility that she was self-medicating. It is relatively easy to purchase medications without a prescription in Mexico.]*

Adding this new information into the picture helped us to formulate another possible problem; the medication Maria had bought in Mexico has been documented to cause problems with weight gain and gastrointestinal problems in some nursing babies.[3]

---

[3] Chambers CD, Anderson PO, Thomas RG, Dick LM, Felix RJ, Johnson KA, Jones KL. Weight gain in infants breastfed by mothers who take fluoxetine. *Peds* 104(5):e61; 1999.

Hale TW, Shum S, Grossberg M. Fluoxetine toxicity in a breastfed infant. *Clin Pediatr* 40(12): 681–4; 2001.

Lester BM, Cucca J, Andreozzi L, Flanagan P, Oh W. Possible association between fluoxetine hydrochloride and colic in an infant. *J Am Acad Child Adolesc Pyschiatry* 32(6):1253–5; 1993.

Level 6—Generate and Prioritize Solutions and Plans for Interventions

The class generated the following list of solutions, which were prioritized in consultation with Maria:

- Pediatric referral re: concerns about Isabel's blood levels of antidepressant, identify growth needs, possible referral to pediatric gastroenterology and growth and development clinic (We were fortunate to have a pediatric clinician from the hospital participating in the class who volunteered to fast track the pediatric referral. She was able to schedule an appointment for the next day with a senior clinician who would be able to facilitate other referrals as needed. This may alleviate another problem: lack of continuity of pediatric care, and perhaps less clarity of the "big picture" of Isabel's growth and development caused by rotation of clinicians.)

- Medical referral for Maria to evaluate medication needs and possibility of anemia

- Schedule an immediate appointment for Maria to meet with her prior counselor

Level 7—Reconcile Prioritized Solutions and Planned Interventions with Problems

The solutions and interventions do not directly correlate with the problems of inadequate milk intake and/or production. A proposal was made to increase feedings to 10 times daily, or substitute feedings with milk expression. Maria stated that she would be willing to nurse Isabel more often, or to hand express her milk (she stated that she was not interested in pumping).

Level 8—Evaluate Solutions and Interventions

Lourdes agreed to follow-up with us all regarding Maria and Isabel's progress. One month later, she contacted us to report that Isabel's antidepressant levels had been found to be twice the therapeutic range for an adult, while Maria's levels were below the therapeutic range. Her internist told her to stop taking that antidepressant, and prescribed another considered safer for a nursing infant. Isabel had been seen by the pediatric and gastroenterology clinics. She had gained almost a pound over the course of the month, so an appointment had not been scheduled with the growth and development clinic. It was unclear whether the weight gain was due to increased feeding, or the cessation of the antidepressant. Maria told Lourdes that Isabel seemed happier, and more robust. "She said that she spends much more time playing with her siblings, or by herself on the floor."

Maria also told Lourdes that her depression had relieved a bit, but she was dealing with a new problem: a wave of guilt over what the medication had been doing to her baby. "She's dealing with such a heavy load of work, worry, and guilt," Lourdes shared. "I'm keeping my fingers crossed for her."

Thoughts

This case provides an excellent example of out-of-the-box thinking (or "out of the bra" in lactation care situations). Did the thought of self-medication for Maria's depression occur to you? It is so important to pay attention to the clues that stand out for us—the words, body language, tone of voice—that catch our attention by their intensity or that seem out of proportion to the situation. How did Tina know to ask about self-medication? She couldn't put her finger on it, except that there was something about Maria's tone when she spoke of not needing the doctor to take care of her. It is important for clinicians to build and hone their listening and observation skills, extending these skills like virtual antennae toward clients, scanning for clues. When circumstances trigger the counselor's "antennae," she should ask for more information about them, thinking like a detective. We cannot possibly imagine all of what any other individual might be thinking, doing, or feeling; however, we can open ourselves to the possibility that there are contributing factors we will not encounter if we keep our thinking in the box.

Further Reading

Schein E. *Process Consultation, Volume I.* Reading, MA: Addison-Wesley Publishing Company; 1988.
Schon DA. *The Reflective Practitioner: How Professionals Think in Action.* New York: Basic Books; 1983.

Discussion Questions

1. Look back over the questions asked by the participants to Ashley or Maria. How many of them are closed-ended questions (questions that can be answered with a yes, a no, or another single word)? How many of them are open-ended questions (questions that require a longer answer)? How is the information that is gathered different

when the question is open versus closed? Choose three closed-ended questions asked to one of the mothers and rephrase it as an open-ended question. How do you think the mother's answer would have been different?

2. What questions make you curious about what the participant was thinking? Can you identify other problems that people might have been formulating? What other problems could you formulate from the symptoms presented?

3. What answers made you want to ask the mother for further information or clarification? What questions do you find yourself wanting to ask her? Why?

Chapter 3

Assessment

*"Look at everything as though you were
seeing it for the first time or the last time."*
—BETTY SMITH, NOVELIST (1896–1972)

The case studies in this chapter focus on the importance of Level 2, assessment, and the value of assessment in the consulting process. The case studies in this chapter include abbreviated assessment reports. Assessment may include

- The physical characteristics of the mother, the baby, and the feeding
- Psychosocial, behavioral, and educational findings
- The relationships and interactions observed
- Diagnostic and other tests
- Anthropometric data
- The observation of artifacts such as pacifiers, the appearance of stool and milk, nipple shields, and other comfort devices
- Milk expression
- Information obtained from other practitioners
- Relevant documents

Although other care providers may have assessed the baby carefully, the assessment of the feeding represents an opportunity to observe the baby in a performance activity. The feeding assessment requires careful and critical observation of the baby's feeding cues, pre-feeding behaviors, and response to the feeding, as well as the ability to transfer milk—a complex, integrated activity.

It's important to have experience with normal infants so that the consultant is able to assess the difference between expected and unexpected findings.

Katrina & Zack

Katrina was a regular participant of a weekly support group at the Center. One day she called to ask for a few minutes to speak with us. We agreed to meet with her immediately after group later that same day.

> *"Wow," we greeted her and her adorable two-month-old baby. "Zack has really grown!"*
>
> *"Yes," she grinned. "He's over 10 pounds now. And does he love to nurse!"*
>
> *"How can we help you, Katrina?"*
>
> *"Well, you know that I really believe in nursing. I don't know if I can keep doing it, though."*
>
> *"Can you tell us more about that?"*
>
> *"I think he's enjoying it too much. He spends a lot of time at the beginning of each feeding licking my nipple, smiling at it, lapping around it. It takes forever for him to get down to business."*
>
> *"How long do you think he spends nosing around before he latches on?"*
>
> *"About a minute or two, probably, but it feels longer. My milk lets down now, and we both get soaked before he gets on."*
>
> *"And when he does get latched on, what happens then?"*
>
> *"He nurses for about 10 minutes and then falls off. I burp him then, and change his diaper if he needs to be*

changed, and put him to the other side. Then he starts the licking stuff all over again."

"Babies are all so different. It sounds like he has a long familiarization phase to his feeding pattern. You know, Anna has done some research on this, and has found that babies who are allowed to complete their familiarization phase before latching are less likely to have mothers with extremely sore nipples."[1]

"Really!" she exclaimed. "I didn't even know that there was a name for what he does. I honestly thought it was a little weird—you know, sensual—but you're telling me it's biological. Awesome!"

"It helps you to know that it's something all babies do."

"Yes, you bet."

"It might be helpful to think of the difference between a gourmet and a gourmand, a picky eater, and an eat-to-live eater. Imagine how each would react to a fine meal. The gourmet would take in the presentation, the aroma, the texture, roll the food and wine around in his mouth, before chewing and swallowing. He would then start all over again with the next bite, appreciating each morsel that he consumes. The gourmand would dive in with great gusto, devouring everything robustly, while the picky eater would push the food around on the plate before deciding if he would try any of it. The eat-to-live eater would consume the amount of food he thought necessary to cover his caloric and nutrient needs, and then push away from the table. Where would you place Zack on this line?"

"Oh, definitely on the gourmet end," she proudly exclaimed. "What a great image! I can't wait to tell it to his grandparents, who are great food snobs! They haven't been supportive of breastfeeding at all."

---

[1] Blair ALC. *Sore Nipples and Breastfeeding: Assessment of the Relationship Between Positioning and Pain.* Ann Arbor, MI: UMI Company; 2003.

Lisa & Jerome

A call came in one morning from a former student, Julie, on the West Coast. She was concerned about a good friend, Lisa, who had moved to a city in New England and had recently given birth to a healthy term boy. She was having trouble breastfeeding, mostly with weight gain. Although the friend was "nursing all the time," the baby was almost three weeks old and not back up to birth weight. The baby's physician was firm about switching to formula at the next visit (in two days) if a substantial amount of weight had not been gained between weeks two and three. Julie felt that her ability to help Lisa with long-distance phone support was limited. Lisa had told Julie that she had visited a lactation consultant several times but Lisa was still concerned about her baby's growth. Julie was afraid the news was not going to be good at the next weigh-in. Julie was worried that things were not getting better and she wondered if we would see Lisa. Julie had talked to Lisa and she was willing to drive to see us.

As it turned out, we were traveling to a hospital only a few miles from where Lisa lived and could visit her on the way home. When we arrived at the mother's home she was about to nurse. The baby had the classic appearance of an underfed baby: scrawny, lethargic, and frowning.

We talked with Lisa for a few minutes and asked questions about her pregnancy and birth. She reported no problems during this, her first pregnancy. She had an epidural and gave birth vaginally after pushing for 1½ hours. The baby (Jerome) weighed 8 pounds 4 ounces at birth.

She told us that both she and Jerome's father were horribly allergic and she was devoted to the idea of no formula in order to decrease his chances of having the problems with allergies that they both had.

Jerome roomed in with her and was an avid feeder in the hospital. She stayed for 24 hours and then had a visiting nurse visit her and Jerome at home. Her milk wasn't "in" when the nurse came and Jerome didn't nurse during the two-hour visit. Her milk "came in" on the fourth day.

She was never engorged but Jerome started having 3–5 wet diapers a day and yellow stool at least once a day starting on day 5. Sometimes the amount of stool was more than other times. Lisa told us that although she had a pacifier to use in the car, she never had to use it.

She told us that she was shocked at the first pediatric checkup at 5 days that Jerome was the same as his discharge weight, 7 pounds 7 ounces. At 10 days he was

7 pounds 8 ounces. She has continued to bring Jerome in for weight checks but now at 22 days she's afraid he still hasn't gained enough.

Lisa also noticed that Jerome's feeding cues were happening less often so she had started to feed him at least every 1½ hours on Julie's advice. The feedings lasted about 40 minutes or longer.

Lisa fed Jerome on both breasts at each feeding. The lactation consultant encouraged her to pump in between feedings in order to increase her supply and she tried to do this, too. The problem was that the time in between feedings was only about a half hour or so and she needed to go to the bathroom, throw in a load of wash, and eat. She did pump "sometimes," and usually could collect about an ounce or so in 15 minutes. Her pump was one she had bought in anticipation of her return to work.

After weighing Jerome on a scale with breast milk intake function, we observed Lisa breastfeeding Jerome in their usual place, her bed, in their usual position, side-lying. Lisa told us that her hemorrhoids had been so painful after pushing for so long that this position was the most comfortable for her at first. Now that her hemorrhoids were tamed, she really enjoyed the snuggling time and found the position restful since she was nursing "almost all the time."

Lisa's left breast was pyramid-shaped with no unusual attributes. We observed that Jerome opened his mouth as he neared Lisa's everted nipple on her left breast, latched on, and sucked. We counted the suck to swallow ratio as high as 20 sucks to 1 swallow with some variation to 8 sucks to 1 swallow. There was no lower suck to swallow ratio observed. Jerome's bottom lip was flanged appropriately, no cheek dimples noted, and nose and chin were placed close to the nipple. He was rotated toward the breast and suckled continuously for 20 minutes. When Lisa ended the nursing on the left side we assessed her nipple. The nipple was everted and appeared not damaged or reddened; there were no white lines indicating compression.

Lisa told us that she usually broke suction, rolled over, and then nursed on the other side. Given the high suck–swallow ratio we had observed, we were not surprised when the after feed weight indicated that no measureable amount of milk had been transferred.

Level 1—History

The history doesn't give us much in the way of clues. Lisa's pregnancy seems uneventful. She reports seeing colostrum during her pregnancy and even had wetness in her bra (Lactogenesis I) and the change to transitional milk (Lactogenesis II) is reported to have happened on the fourth day. Also, her lochia is creamy (suggesting complete delivery of the placenta). She has some milk and has been able to pump a small amount. Jerome's stools are yellow, and he has a few wet diapers and at least one stool a day. Jerome has been checked repeatedly by the pediatrician and his mother reports that he is normal except for growth.

Level 2—Assessment

Lisa's left nipple is everted; her breast is cone shaped; there are a few visible veins. Jerome is able to latch onto the breast correctly, maintains color and energy throughout the feeding, and moves his mouth appropriately. His hands remain clenched throughout the feeding. The suck to swallow ratio is high, indicating a low milk flow. Jerome does not indicate the beginning of feedings by cue or end the feedings by letting go. Also, the before and after weights indicate little-to-no milk transfer. The nursing pattern is one of almost constant feeding.

Level 3—Symptoms

- Inadequate weight gain (but Jerome hasn't lost any additional weight)
- Inadequate milk transfer as indicated by the high suck to swallow ratio and the milk intake as measured on the digital scale

Level 4—Problem Formulation

- Problem 1: Inadequate weight gain for three weeks
- Problem 2: Low milk supply and/or inadequate let-down/milk-ejection reflex

Level 5—Reconcile the History, Assessment, Symptoms, and Problems

There isn't anything in the mother's history that helps us know why Lisa would have a low milk supply and/or problems with her let-down reflex. We cannot go on to Level 6 (make a plan for intervention) until we can get a better understanding of the connection between the history, assessment, symptoms, and what we think might be the problem.

Because we can't complete Level 5 at this point with any confidence, we need to delve further into the history, assessment, and symptom levels again.

> *We asked Lisa to nurse on the right breast, first recording Jerome's before feeding weight. As soon as she began getting ready we observed that her right breast was two-to-three times larger than her left breast and conical, with visible veins in a symmetrical pattern. [Color Plate 3-1]*
>
> *Jerome latched on as he had onto the left breast and began suckling in an 8:1 suck to swallow ratio. After a minute or so, a pattern of 3:1 and 2:1 sucks to swallows occurred for about three minutes. Jerome then went back to the pattern of 8 sucks to 1 swallow. We asked Lisa to stroke her breast (alternate massage). She stroked from the back of the breast to the front with her left hand. Each time she performed alternate massage the suck to swallow ratio went down to 3:1 or 2:1. We pointed out the effect of massage on the suck to swallow pattern.*

Alternate massage is an effective way to increase the rate of milk flow. There is some interest in the idea that the rapidity of milk removal is an important influence on the rate of milk synthesis.[2] If Lisa's low milk supply is being delivered slowly this could inhibit the volume of milk she makes.

> *Lisa ended the feeding by breaking suction after 20 minutes. According to the after feeding weight, Jerome had taken in 1.6 ounces. [Color Plate 3-2]*
>
> *We asked Lisa about her discrepant breast size. She said that they had been that way ever since she could remember . . . . it took a lot of tissues to stuff the left cup of her bra! We asked her if the hospital staff had compared her two breasts. She said that she didn't think anyone had watched her nurse on both sides before today. We asked if she had been born prematurely or if she had a chest tube implanted as a child. She told us that she had been a preemie and her*

---

[2] Creagan MD, Hartmann PE. Computerized breast measurement from conception to weaning: Clinical implication. *J Hum Lact.* 15(2):89; 1999.

mother told her to never smoke because of all the lung prob-
lems she had in the hospital. As to the specific question
about the chest tube, she didn't know. Sadly, her mother
had passed away four years before.

Level 1—History

We can now add to the history the possibility that Lisa's left breast has
not developed normally possibly because of the placement of a chest
tube in the area of that breast as a premature infant.

Level 2—Assessment

We now add the right breast to our assessment. The right breast looks
identical in shape to the left breast but is two to three times bigger.
There are many more veins visible and they are seen all over the
breast. The nipple is everted. Jerome is able to transfer 1.6 ounces of
milk from the right breast as evidenced by before and after weights
with a digital scale with breast milk intake function.

Level 3—Symptoms

(The symptom list doesn't change)

- Inadequate weight gain (but Jerome hasn't lost any additional
  weight)
- Inadequate milk transfer as indicated by the high suck-to-swallow
  ratio and the milk intake as measured on the digital scale

Level 4—Problem Formulation

(The problem list doesn't change)

- Problem 1: Inadequate weight gain for three weeks
- Problem 2: Low milk supply and/or inadequate let-down/milk-
  ejection reflex

Level 5—Reconcile the History, Assessment, Symptoms, and Problems

Now that we have compared the two breasts and observed the difference in feeding and milk transfer, the reconciliation can take shape.
Lisa's left breast is functioning marginally, if at all, and her right breast
may be functioning normally, but is not producing sufficient milk to

support Jerome's growth. Jerome, therefore, is spending half of his time nursing without getting much milk. He has maintained his weight, but has not gained as expected.

Now that we have been able to negotiate Level 5, we can move on to Level 6 with solutions and plans that emerge from Levels 1 to 5. We still have unanswered questions. Will Lisa be able to increase her milk supply in her right breast in order to produce and deliver enough milk for an adequate weight gain? Will she be able to do this fast enough to avoid formula as is her desire? If Jerome needs to be supplemented, what are the choices for nutrition and delivery?

Level 6—Generate and Prioritize Solutions and Plans for Interventions

We couldn't eliminate either of the two problems because they are interrelated and equally significant, but Jerome's weight gain is the first priority.

- Plan for Problem 1: Jerome will gain weight (catch up) and grow normally. He will have gained an average of at least one ounce per day by his next pediatric checkup.

We can estimate the amount of milk Jerome needs by multiplying his current weight (7 pounds 7 ounces) by 2.7. The number 2.5 is used in the early weeks for babies who don't need to catch up. These numbers are only approximate and need to be continually evaluated, but they are good as a starting point. So, 7 pounds 7 ounces is approximately 7.5 pounds times 2.7, equalling approximately 20.25 ounces to be consumed in 24 hours. We don't know if we observed a typical feeding with a transfer of about 1.6 ounces on the right breast and nothing on the left, but if that is the average, and Lisa nurses 10 times a day, that's only 16 ounces—not enough.

In order to ensure that Jerome is getting enough milk, we recommend that Lisa have a digital scale with breast milk function at home and use it to record feedings. She will need to write down the amounts that Jerome takes in with the goal of a minimum of 20.25 ounces today, increasing each day as his weight increases. Is Lisa willing (and able) to do this? We think so and she thinks so.

What if Jerome doesn't start to gain by the next pediatric weight check? Lisa can ask the physician to prescribe donor breast milk from a human milk bank if she doesn't want to use formula. If additional nourishment is needed, we will help her to feed Jerome at her breast with an at-breast feeding tube system; because Jerome is able to make a seal and suckle, the at-breast feeding tube system should work well.

- Plan for Problem 2: Increase Lisa's milk production on the right breast in order to meet Jerome's catch-up and growth needs.

If Lisa's right breast is functioning normally, she should be able to make and deliver enough milk in her right breast for Jerome to grow adequately.[3] One positive indicator is that her current production and delivery on her right breast is close to what Jerome needs, but because he has been nursing half of the time on what seems to be a low functioning breast, sufficient milk is not being transferred.

Also on the positive side, Jerome is still an avid nurser. Although many chronically underfed infants become sleepy and apathetic, Jerome is willing to spend a great deal of time at the breast and is able to transfer almost as much milk as he needs. We believe that if there were additional milk he would be able to take it.

Our suggestion to Lisa was that she work to build her milk supply in her right breast by letting Jerome feed only on her right breast, using alternate massage when his suck to swallow ratio increased over 3:1. Because he wasn't indicating when to feed, she should continue to nurse every hour or so for 15 to 20 minutes, taking before and after weights.

> *Lisa was willing to limit nursings to her right breast, use alternate massage, and weigh Jerome before and after feedings. A neighbor offered to drive to a pharmacy in a nearby town to pick up a digital scale for Lisa that afternoon. Before we left, Lisa nursed again on her right breast and Jerome transferred approximately 2.1 ounces. Lisa's neighbor arrived with the scale just as we were leaving.*

> *When we checked in with Lisa the next afternoon she told us that Jerome had taken 22 ounces in the past 24 hours according to the sum of before and after weights. She told us that at the end of his last nursing he let go of the nipple and relaxed his hands.*

> *When we talked to Lisa right after the next weigh-in, Jerome was 2 ounces above birth weight and on his way to an adequate weight gain.*

[3] Huggins KE, Petok ES, Mireles O. Markers of lactation insufficiency: A study of 34 mothers. In: Auerbach K. *Current Issues in Clincical Lactation 2002.* Sudbury, MA: Jones and Bartlett Publishers; 2002.

Here is a review of our assessment:

Assessment of Baby

Attributes	Observed	Comments
Infant state	Yes	Drowsy, continues to be drowsy throughout the feeding, then deep sleep. No other states observed.
Sufficient energy	Yes, but marginal	Indicates urgency.
Flexion	Yes	
Appropriate reaction to stimulation	Yes	
Ability to orient to breast, concentrate and work at feeding	Yes	
Becomes more organized when soothed	No	Baby never needed to be soothed during observation.
Intact suck, gag, and rooting reflexes	Yes	
Coordinated suck, swallow, breathe	Yes	
Symmetry	Yes	
Motor activity appropriate for the physiologic state	Yes	But limited observation. No crying noted.
Expressive face with yawn or cry	Not observed	
Loud, lusty cry	Not observed	
Ability to orient to breast and nipple	Yes	

Assessment of Mother

Attributes	Observed	Comments
Symmetrical breasts	No	Right breast was 2–3 times larger than left.
Compressible breast tissue	Yes	
Visible veins with an overall pattern	Right breast only	Left breast had scant venation compared to right.
Intact, smooth epithelium on the breast	Yes	

continues

Assessment of Mother (continued)

Attributes	Observed	Comments
Montgomery glands visible on the areola	Yes	
Evenly pigmented, wrinkled nipple surface	Yes	
Presence of milk	Yes in right breast only	No milk observed or transferred from left breast.
Patent milk ducts in the breast and nipple	Yes	Droplets visible in right breast only.
Evidence of innervation of the breast and nipple	Yes	Nipples evert in response to stimulus.
Rapid removal of milk	No	Alternate massage increased milk removal.
Everted, tubular shaped nipples	Yes	
Intact neuromuscular ability to support infant	Yes	
Maternal hormones	No	Mother reports normal levels of thyroid hormones, blood iron. She also reports normal breast changes prenatally and postpartum.
Other physiologic indicators		History of maternal prematurity and possible chest tube in infancy.
Education of mother related to breastfeeding	Yes	Mother is knowledgeable and seeks information appropriately.
Behavior of mother related to breastfeeding	Yes	Mother is willing to nurse frequently and change her behavior to increase baby's weight gain and her milk supply.

Assessment of the Feeding

Attributes	Observed	Comments
Feeding cues	No	
Gape	Yes	
Wide open mouth	Yes	
Nipple position	Yes	No dimples, smooth cheek line, no compression on nipple at the end of the feeding.

continues

Assessment of Feeding (continued)

Attributes	Observed	Comments
Forming and maintaining the seal	Yes	
Nursing dynamic	Yes	2:1, 3:1, and 8:1 modified by alternate massage on the right breast; 20:1 and 8:1 on the left.
Releasing the breast, ending the feed	No	Mother ended the feeding after 20 minutes on each side by breaking suction with her finger.

Assessment of Artifacts

Attributes	Observed	Comments
Pump(s)	No	Mother reports pumping 1 ounce occasionally.
Breast and nipple comfort devices	No	Mother reports that she does not use any.
Creams or soothing agents	No	Mother reports that she does not use any.
Nipple shield	No	Mother reports she does not use one.
At-breast feeding system	No	Not used.
Bottles and artificial nipples	No	Not used.
Non-breast milk feeds	No	Not used.
Cups and other feeders	No	Not used.
Pacifier	No	Not used.
Galactogogues	No	Not used.
Drugs and medications	No	Mother reports she does not use OTC, recreational, or prescription drugs or herbs. She does take prenatal vitamins.
Diapers	Yes	Quarter-sized yellow stool stain.

Level 7—Reconcile Prioritized Solutions and Planned Interventions with Problems

The proposed solutions and interventions appear to appropriate for the problems.

Level 8—Evaluate Solutions and Interventions

As we review this case, it's clear that the finding that the left breast was virtually nonfunctional is the key to the development of a unique and directed plan. Several health care workers examined and/or assisted Lisa during the peripartum period. Unfortunately none of them picked up on the clue of discrepant breast size. It is not our intention to pass judgment on these individual care providers—none of us are perfect. The problem might have been solved sooner had it been discovered by her prenatal care provider during physical examination, or in the hospital by a nurse, physician, or lactation consultant, or in the community by a pediatrician, pediatric office staff member, visiting nurse, or lactation consultant.

The intervention of building up her milk supply on the right breast evolved from Level 5 of the process: recognizing that we were not able to reconcile the history, assessment, symptoms, and problems after observing Jerome nursing on the left breast. The use of a digital scale with breast milk intake function was invaluable for both the assessment (Level 2) and the intervention (Level 6).

Shawna, Mike, & Colin

In this case we can also see the importance of a complete assessment.

One of our local pediatricians called on a Friday morning. Shawna and her baby Colin were in the office. Colin was 15 days old and still at discharge weight. Shawna wanted to continue exclusively breastfeeding but the pediatrician wanted a complete feeding assessment before making a decision about formula supplementation. Shawna and Colin could come over to the Center for Breastfeeding for a feeding assessment if we could see them right away.

The Center for Breastfeeding provides consultations, classes, and telephone support during office hours, 9–5, Monday through Friday. About 10 percent of our contacts are directly with care providers, midwives, visiting nurses, pediatricians, obstetricians, and other lactation care providers. The other 90 percent of our contacts are with mothers and their babies, often, as in this case, by referral. We also make home visits when they are warranted. Sometimes one of the Center lactation consultants might coordinate a home visit at the same time as the visiting nurse. We are also asked to go to medical offices to consult on cases. We work closely with the USDA's Special Supplemental Nutrition Program for Women, Infants and Children (WIC) program to provide support to their peer counselors and nutritionists. Because we are in an area with geographical challenges (rural islands, one hundred miles from either Boston or Providence and their tertiary health care facilities) and without public transportation, we are fortunate to have the support of our local airline, that donates vouchers so that we can fly to rural areas to make home visits. In this case, Shawna and Colin had a car and could drive to our site.

Shawna and baby Colin arrived along with Colin's dad, Mike, in just a few minutes. Both Shawna and Mike were visibly upset. Shawna cried several times while they were with us and Mike sat next to her on the couch with his arm around her shoulder. Colin slept in his car seat as they told us about the pregnancy and birth.

Colin was born via cesarean 15 days earlier. Shawna had high blood pressure toward the end of her pregnancy but otherwise no problems. Her breasts increased in size and she noticed colostrum leaking in the last trimester. The birth really "threw her for a loop," according to Mike. After being in labor for practically two days, she had the cesarean because of "failure to progress." She felt terrible after the surgery, throwing up and in a great deal of pain. The pain medication made her sick and sleepy and Colin didn't really nurse well until just before they left the hospital.

Shawna told us that she felt like a failure all the way around and now breastfeeding wasn't working out either. Mike was convinced that breast milk was the best for Colin. Shawna had had plenty of milk starting on day 5. She soaks bra pads, sleeps in a milky wet bed, and sprays milk all over the place. "He gets these little milk drops all over his head." They couldn't understand why he wasn't gaining.

Colin weighed 8 pounds 11 ounces at birth and his discharge weight was 8 pounds 2 ounces. Now, on day 15, he weighs 8 pounds 3 ounces. Shawna nurses Colin 8 times a day at least, according to the parents. If he sleeps for more than 3 hours they wake him up and he's usually happy to nurse. Colin usually nurses on both breasts.

Colin began chewing on his fists as we spoke. Mike responded to the feeding cue spontaneously and immediately took Colin out of the car seat and got him ready to nurse. We weighed Colin prior to the nursing. As soon as Colin was 1 inch from his mother's nipple he gaped and started rooting on his hand. He opened his mouth wide, grasped the breast well behind the base of the nipple, and began suckling. The suck to swallow ratio was 8:1 at first, but after 30 seconds he settled into a good rocker motion with 2:1 and 1:1 sucks to swallows predominating.

Shawna broke suction after 10 minutes. At this point Colin was no longer nursing avidly. He went to the second breast, nursed another 7 minutes with periodic 1:1 and 2:2 suck to swallow ratios and released the nipple to end the feed, his hands relaxed. He had transferred about 3 ounces according to the post weight. A good feed!

Level 1—History

Shawna reports that she had normal breast changes in pregnancy and her "milk came in" on the fourth day. Colin got off to a slow start but really began to nurse well around the time Shawna had a more abundant milk supply. The parents tell us that they nurse 8 times a day, at least every 3 hours for between 15 and 20 minutes. Colin has 1 or 2 yellow stools at least every day or every other day and about 3–5 wet diapers a day.

Level 2—Assessment

Shawna's breasts are symmetrical and have obvious veins. The nipples were everted before and after the feeding with no distortion or compression lines. Colin showed feeding cues and rooting prior to the feeding, and gaped, latched, and nursed well on both sides. He took himself off of the second breast spontaneously and his hands were relaxed. Colin transferred 3 ounces according to our before and after weights. If the feeding we had seen was typical, Colin was getting about 24 ounces a day. Using the calculation of 2.5–2.7 ounces needed per pound, Colin needs between 20 and 22 ounces a day. He should be gaining by leaps and bounds, but he isn't. His stools and wet diapers are indicative of inadequate feeds. We would expect more than 3 stools a day at a minimum, with many well-fed infants stooling at every feed. Wet diapers are difficult to assess, especially since Colin wore paper diapers known for their absorbent construction.

Level 3—Symptoms

- Inadequate weight gain

Level 4—Problem Formulation

Thoughts

As we ponder how to formulate this problem, we asked ourselves a series of questions. Where is the problem? Did Shawna and Colin just get off to a slow start? We felt confident that Colin could transfer sufficient milk and that Shawna could deliver enough milk; were they just catching up? Because we couldn't articulate a problem based on the history and assessment, we needed to continue to gather information.

First, we called the pediatrician and reported what we found and asked if we could defer a formal report until Monday afternoon. We would send a scale home with Shawna and Mike and ask them to keep a feeding log over the weekend, and come back to see us Monday morning. Then we would have more information and they could go back to the pediatrician after meeting with us, if needed.

We were working with a few possibilities, which could be sorted out over the weekend. The first, of course, was that Colin was on the verge of gaining but that he and Shawna had gotten off to a slow start. If this was the case, he should gain an ounce or two over the weekend. The second possibility we were considering was that Shawna *thought* she was nursing eight times a day, but, in fact, it was really only five or six times. She told us that she was always wet with milk, soaking bra pads, soaking the bed, and soaking her sweatshirts. Her leaking may have relieved any compression on her milk-making cells.

> *We taught Shawna and Mike how to use the digital scale. We provided them with a feeding, wet diaper, and stool log and instructions to make notes about the feeding—time of day, how long it lasted, before and after weights, etc. We would be calling them over the weekend to see how things were going and they would come into the Center on Monday morning.*
>
> *When Shawna and Mike were called on Saturday, they reported that everything was going well, no problems so far. On Sunday they were excited. They had discovered that although Colin's weights indicated transfers of 2.5 ounces to 3 ounces per feeding when Shawna sat up to nurse (as she had on the couch in the Center) he only transferred 1 ounce or less if she nursed him lying down. Because of how tired she was and the painful after effects of the cesarean, Shawna was nursing lying down at least half the time!*
>
> *Mike, Shawna, and Colin were at the Center when we opened on Monday morning. They started telling us their story before even taking their coats off. By Sunday morning they had seen the pattern emerging: Good transfers sitting up, much less milk lying down. "So I started nursing only sitting up of course!" Shawna told us. When Shawna nursed lying down to show us, we observed that Colin had a very poor seal. Milk dribbled out of his*

mouth especially on the side closest to the mattress. "No wonder my bed was so wet!" Shawna was making enough milk, but the transfer to Colin was poor in a lying down position. We now could formulate our problem.[4]

Level 4—Problem Formulation

- Inadequate milk transfer when nursing lying down

We can now go on to attempting Level 5.

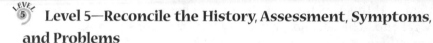

Level 5—Reconcile the History, Assessment, Symptoms, and Problems

Colin is gaining poorly in spite of our assessment that he is able to transfer 3 ounces. The parents discover that he transfers 1 ounce or less when nursed lying down. Since he is nursing lying down for about half of the feedings, this would account for the inadequate weight gain.

Level 6—Generate and Prioritize Solutions and Plans for Interventions

The plan follows from the problem and the assessment: Nurse Colin in the position that he transfers the maximum amount of milk. In Shawna and Colin's case, this is in a sitting up position. Shawna is willing to do this. We offer to help her achieve a better lying down position. She tells us that she just wants to see Colin gaining for right now. She'll come back another time if she wants to get better at side lying.

Level 7—Reconcile Prioritized Solutions and Planned Interventions with Problems

We feel comfortable that the solutions and interventions reconcile well with the problem.

Level 8—Evaluate Solutions and Interventions

We faxed our report to the pediatric office. Shawna, Colin, and Mike left our office for a weight check. They called to tell us the results later

---

[4] It's important to note that in other cases we have seen the opposite: babies who nurse well lying down and not so well in other positions. The mother's comfort, the shape of her breasts, and so on, could be factors as well as baby factors such as birth trauma or anatomical features. Whatever the position, the baby must have a clear airway and the most efficient transfer of milk.

that day, 8 pounds 6 ounces, a gain of an ounce a day since their Friday visit. They would keep the scale at home and monitor feedings for another week, and go to the pediatric office again for a weight check on Wednesday and Friday.

Because Shawna and Mike participated in solving their breast-feeding problem, their confidence in themselves as parents and their confidence in Shawna's ability to nurse Colin increased. This was especially important after the feelings of failure Shawna expressed related to her pregnancy and birth.

Here's a review of our assessment.

Assessment of Baby

Attributes	Observed	Comments
Infant state	All states	
Sufficient energy	Yes	
Flexion	Yes	
Appropriate reaction to stimulation	Yes	
Ability to orient to breast, concentrate, and work at feeding	Yes	
Becomes more organized when soothed	Yes	
Intact suck, gag, and rooting reflex	Yes	
Coordinated suck, swallow, breathe	Yes	
Symmetry	Yes	
Motor activity appropriate for the physiologic state	Yes	
Expressive face with yawn or cry	Yes	
Loud, lusty cry	Yes	
Ability to orient to breast and nipple	Yes	

Assessment of Mother

Attributes	Observed	Comments
Symmetrical breasts	Yes	
Compressible breast tissue	Yes	
Visible veins with an overall pattern	Yes	
Intact, smooth epithelium on the breast	Yes	
Montgomery glands visible on the areola	Yes	
Evenly pigmented, wrinkled nipple surface	Yes	
Presence of milk	Yes	
Patent milk ducts in the breast and nipple	Yes	
Evidence of innervation of the breast and nipple	Yes	Nipples became more erect when touched by Colin's hand or mouth.
Rapid removal of milk	Yes	Suck–swallow 2:1 or 1:1, transfer of 3 ounces by pre- and post-weights.
Everted, tubular shaped nipples	Yes	
Intact neuromuscular ability to support infant	Yes	
Maternal hormones	No	Observed spraying milk, wet bra pads, and transfer of milk.
Other physiologic indicators	No	Shawna was not anemic at the end of pregnancy, her last blood test showed normal thyroid levels.
Education of mother related to breastfeeding	Yes	
Behavior of mother related to breastfeeding	Yes	Mother and father respond to feeding cues, willing to work towards solving problems.

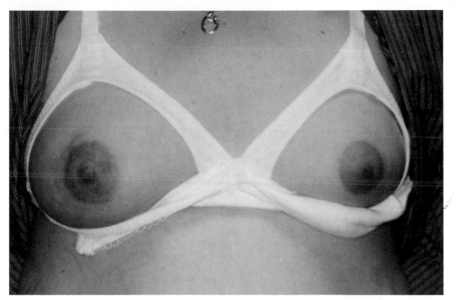

COLOR PLATE 3–1 Assymetrical breasts with normal milk production

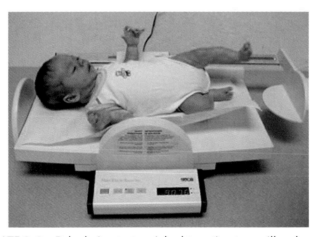

COLOR PLATE 3–2 Baby being test weighed to estimate a milk volume

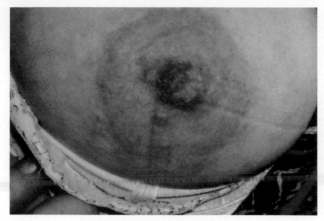

COLOR PLATE 4–1 Fissured, abraded nipple before feeding

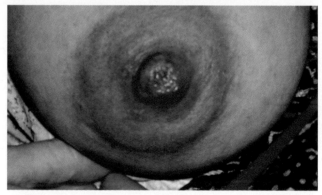

COLOR PLATE 4–2 Fissured nipple after feeding

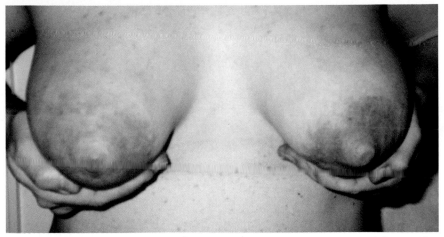

COLOR PLATE 4–3 Raynaud's phenomenon: Normal appearance of the nipples before feeding

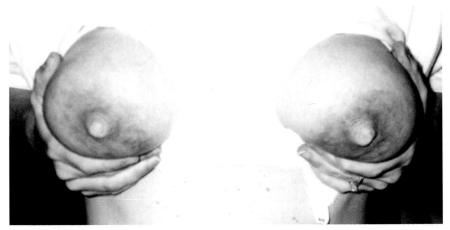

COLOR PLATE 4–4 Raynaud's phenomenon: Blanching of the nipples immediately after feeding

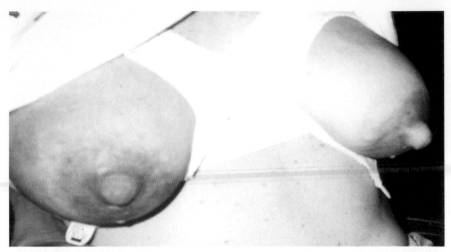

COLOR PLATE 4–5 Raynaud's phenomenon: Appearance of nipples just after pumping

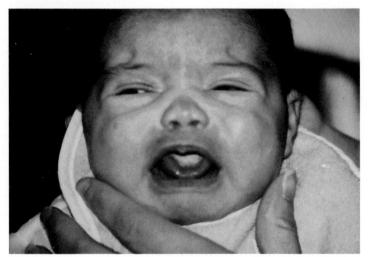

COLOR PLATE 4–6 Baby with visible thrush on tongue

Assessment of the Feeding

Attributes	Observed	Comments
Feeding cues	Yes	
Gape	Yes	
Wide open mouth	Yes	
Nipple position	Yes	Colin grasped nipple well back on the areola, nipple was not compressed or malformed at the end of nursing.
Forming and maintaining the seal	Yes, in sitting position	Not in lying down position.
Nursing dynamic	Yes	2:1 and 1:1 observed.
Releasing the breast, ending the feed	Yes	Colin ended the feed on the second breast.

Assessment of Artifacts

Attributes	Observed	Comments
Pump(s)	No	Mother has a pump but has not used it.
Breast and nipple comfort devices	No	Not used according to the mother.
Creams or soothing agents	No	Not used according to the mother.
Nipple shield	No	
At-breast feeding system	No	
Bottles and artificial nipples	No	
Non-breastmilk feeds	No	
Cups and other feeders	No	
Pacifier	No	
Galactogogues	No	
Drugs and medications	No	
Diapers	Yes	At second visit, substantial amount of yellow, seedy stool in wet diaper. Parents report that increased sitting up feedings resulted in more wet diapers and stools.

We can see in these two examples how important it is for each level to build on the others. In the case of Lisa and Jerome, other care providers Lisa had seen did not perform complete assessments; skipping or glossing over any level, in this case the assessment level (2), can lead to wrong, incomplete, or inadequate resolution of breastfeeding problems.

Lisa's breasts were always different sizes; they just weren't assessed in relation to each other. As a result, the solution of pumping had been suggested by another lactation care provider. Pumping did not fit into Lisa's time constraints and did not change the outcome.

In the case of Shawna and Colin, our assessment of a 3-ounce transfer of milk (and the parents' report of nursing at least eight times a day) didn't make sense in relation to Colin's poor weight gain. More assessment was needed and the assessment had to include multiple feedings. Fortunately, Shawna and Mike were willing and able to do this at home. Also, the pediatrician felt comfortable waiting until Monday to make a decision about supplementing Colin. If Colin needed to be supplemented, perhaps Shawna would have begun collecting milk. Our assessment indicated that she had sufficient milk and a functioning letdown. If Colin's condition warranted it, additional feedings of expressed milk would have been started right away.

Further Reading

Cadwell K, Turner-Maffei C, O'Connor B, Blair A. *Maternal and Infant Assessment for Breastfeeding and Human Lactation: A Guide for the Practitioner.* Sudbury, MA: Jones and Bartlett Publishers; 2002.

Lawrence RA, Lawrence RM. *Breastfeeding: A Guide for the Medical Profession.* St. Louis, MO: Mosby, Inc; 1999.

Huggins KE, Petok ES, Mireles O. Markers of lactation insufficiency: A study of 34 mothers. In: Auerbach, K. *Current Issues in Clincical Lactation 2002.* Sudbury, MA: Jones and Bartlett Publishers; 2002.

Rainer C, Gardetto A, Frühwirth M, et al. Breast Deformity in Adolescense as a Result of Pneumothorax Drainage During Neonatal Intensive Care. Pediatrics III (I): 80–86; 2003.

Discussion Questions

1. What do you notice first when completing a breastfeeding assessment? As you review the assessments that are part of this chapter, which of the parameters do you observe routinely? Which of the parameters might you have neglected in the past?

2. Can you think of a case in which a more thorough assessment would have made a difference in the breastfeeding outcome?

3. Can you think of a situation in which the performance activity of breastfeeding might reveal problems with the baby that other assessments might not?

4. Using the information presented in one of the first two case studies in this chapter, complete the eight levels below:

   Level 1—History:

   Level 2—Assessment:

   Level 3—Symptoms:

   - _____
   - _____
   - _____

   Level 4—Problem Formulation:

   - _____
   - _____
   - _____

   Level 5—Reconcile the History, Assessment, Symptoms, and Problems:

   Level 6—Generate and Prioritze Solutions and Plans for Interventions:

   - _____
   - _____
   - _____

Level 7—Reconcile Prioritized Solutions and Planned Interventions with Problems:

Level 8—Evaluate Solutions and Interventions:

Chapter 4

Symptoms Versus Problems

*"We are too accustomed to attribute
to a single cause that which is
the product of several."*

—Justus von Liebig, chemist (1803–1873)

In this chapter we explore the characteristics of symptoms versus problems. Symptoms are described by the mother or noted in the baby or the feeding. Problems are formulated by the consultant and mother together and explain or support the symptoms. Problems are best formulated in a way that allows directed action. The intent of the consultant when formulating problems is that they be solved.

Joan & Miguel

While training health care providers in a midwestern state our hostess Mari, a newly hired public health worker who was also new to the field of breastfeeding, asked if we could make a home visit to her sister, Joan, who had very sore nipples. Joan's baby was now 10 days old. Mari told us that she rented a breast pump for Joan and also bought a double-pumping kit. They were in the trunk of the car when she picked us up at our hotel along with other supplies, such as a tube of breast care cream, two nipple shields, bottles, and bottle nipples she bought at her local pharmacy.

Mari told us that Joan was ready to quit breastfeeding because of her painfully sore nipples, so she hoped to save breastfeeding by starting Joan at pumping and feeding the baby, Miguel, by bottle until Joan's nipples healed. On the way to Joan's house, Mari filled us in on the details, as she knew them. "I told Joan that her nipples would be sore for 7 to 10 days and now that they are still so painful she wants to quit. I've told her how good breastfeeding is for Miguel, but she feels like it hurts too much."

Mari continued, "She just comes back at me that I've never had a baby and I don't know what this is like for her. She told me this afternoon that I've been brainwashed by my new job. We were both fed formula and we turned out okay. I have heard that the latch-on is important. Joan's was checked in the hospital and it's fine."

Mari's newly acquired supplies and the breast pump were possible solutions for the *symptom* of sore nipples; however, interventions should be directed at the *problem* level (4). This is a classic error of novices. We are often asked the question "What do you do for sore nipples?" Our answer is to find out what *problem* is causing the *symptom* of sore nipples and find a solution for that. Because the problem hasn't been determined (we only know a symptom) a unique and directed plan for Joan can't be developed. As a result, the trunk of Mari's car is full of virtually every product she could find at the pharmacy that claimed to be a solution for sore nipples. A good plan for the people who manufacture and sell these products, not such a good plan for the mother with sore nipples.

> *Joan met us at the door of her lovely suburban home. After introductions, we were invited to sit in the living room. We asked Joan about her pregnancy and birth experience. She told us that her pregnancy was perfect. "I felt queasy for a few weeks, but otherwise I had a great pregnancy. The birth was tough, but Mari found a doula for me, and I have to say I'd do that again if I ever have another baby. I labored in a tub of water and didn't need anything except a little Tylenol after he was born."*
>
> *"Mari told me all about the benefits of breastfeeding, but the one that hit me hardest was the idea of getting back into shape faster. Miguel hurt me right from the beginning with his sucking, but everyone told me that my latch was fine*

*and that my nipples would toughen up by 10 days. Well it's
10 days. I'm done. I'll just lose weight by dieting."*

Unfortunately, we have heard this many times before; sore nipples are
the mother's fault, she needs to "toughen up," and that should happen
in some preordained length of time. We examined this in a research
study of more than 90 mothers with sore nipples[1] in cooperation with
the Association of Midwives of Latvia, and found that sore nipples
responded to optimizing the position and the latch. Almost every
mother's sore nipples improved with the intervention of position and
latch changes.

Mari had talked her sister into breastfeeding and was more
invested in preserving breastfeeding than Joan. This is obviously a
source of conflict between the sisters. Joan hadn't had a single pleasurable moment of breastfeeding and the only benefit that resonated
for her, losing weight, was something she knew she could do with diet
and exercise.

> *Mari was impatient to get working on the symptom.
> While we talked, she assembled the breast pump, kit, and
> nipple creams, etc., on Joan's dining room table. "Let's
> just get you pumping. We had an in-service at work from
> the pump company sales woman and I can get this all
> set up. You can pump while your nipples heal, that's
> what the pump company woman told us."*

Taking a look at the levels, let's see where we are.

Level 1—History

Joan had an uneventful pregnancy and a normal birth. Breastfeeding
has been painful from the first nursing and has continued for 10 days.
The pain begins when Miguel starts nursing and hurts during every
feeding.

Level 2—Assessment

We have not observed the mother's breasts, seen the baby, or observed
a nursing. We have the mother's description of pain. On a one-to-five
scale with one being no pain—just tugging and five being the worst
pain ever, Joan says nursing is a five.

---

[1] Cadwell K, Turner-Maffei C, Blair A, Brimdyr K. *Pain Reduction and Treatment of
Sore Nipples in Nursing Mothers.* In press.

Level 3—Symptoms

- Painful, sore nipples during breastfeeding

Level 4—Problem Formulation

Without a more complete assessment, we can't develop a problem list. What we see in this case is that Mari has confused the symptom (Level 3) and the problem (Level 4). She wants to generate solutions to the symptom of sore nipples not to the as yet unknown *problem*. Although a nipple cream or device may be an appropriate tool for our solution, we can't know that from a symptom of sore nipples with a scanty assessment.

We also need to remember that whoever told Joan that she had a great latch did so when Joan was in the hospital, most likely in the colostral phase of lactation. Some babies nurse effectively with high-viscosity, low-volume colostrum but may have problems managing to transfer an abundant flow of milk. Other babies become more organized feeders with an abundant flow. Joan told us that nursing hurt right from the first time. That makes us think that the change in flow from colostrum to transitional milk has nothing to do with her pain.

> We tell Joan that we are happy to try to help her if she'd like, but in order to do this we will need to observe a nursing. She says that it hurts too much, she doesn't want to nurse ever again. She has the formula from her hospital discharge bag that she was going to use tonight, but she'll nurse once more. We tell her that we need to see how Miguel takes the nipple without any suggestions from us. As soon as we have completed our assessment she can stop and we'll talk about what to do next.

> We followed Joan to the nursery. Miguel was fussing in his crib, alternately sucking on his hand and crying. Joan told us that they had been to the pediatrician's office for a weigh-in two days before and Miguel had gained 2 ounces since leaving the hospital. The pediatric nurse practitioner was pleased with Miguel's progress.

> Joan picked Miguel up and competently changed the diaper. She sat in a rocking/gliding chair, put her feet up onto a footstool, and arranged a thick, hard foam pillow on her lap. She settled Miguel on his back on top of the pillow and took her right breast in her left hand and flicked the nipple back and forth across Miguel's lips.

*Her breast appeared to have been compressed by her bra;
bra seams were indented on her breasts. [Color Plate 4-1]
We observed a scab line across the nipple tip from 1:00 to
7:00. Miguel rooted over his left shoulder and still lying on
his back, began to suck, pulling at the nipple. "It hurts! It
really hurts!" We encouraged Joan to break suction. Even
with this brief suckling, Joan's nipple was distorted and
compressed. The scab was gone and a fissure with white
compression lines was observed in its place.*

We were now ready to attempt to formulate the problem, considering
this new information.

 ## Level 2—Assessment

We can add to this level because we've observed a nursing. The baby's
head position and body position were suboptimal. The baby was
unable to correctly place the nipple in his mouth because of his body
position. The damage to Joan's nipple was consistent with repeated
suboptimal positionings for nursing. When we examined Joan's left
nipple, the crack went from 11:00 to 5:00. We asked if she nursed in a
similar position on both breasts. She told us that she did.

 ## Level 3—Symptoms

This level stays almost the same except that we have now observed the
damage to Joan's nipples.

- Painful, fissured, sore nipples

 ## Level 4—Problem Formulation

We can now formulate the problem.

- Suboptimal positioning of the baby at the breast resulting in
  suboptimal positioning of the nipple in the baby's mouth

 ## Level 5—Reconcile the History, Assessment, Symptoms, and Problems

We feel confident that we can reconcile the history of painful, sore, and
cracked nipples from the earliest nursings with the assessment of
Miguel's nursing position and Joan's nipples.

Level 6—Generate and Prioritize Solutions and Plans for Interventions

Joan said that she wants to stop breastfeeding. The interaction of the two sisters indicates that this is a hot button with Joan saying it's over and Mari insistent that Joan continue to breastfeed Miguel.

> We explained to Joan and Mari that we now had a good idea of the problem: Miguel's position at the breast and the placement of her nipple in Miguel's mouth had injured the nipple and was responsible for at least some of the pain. Would Joan be willing to try to nurse one more time, with our help, positioning Miguel in a way that might minimize the discomfort?

Level 7—Reconcile Prioritized Solutions and Planned Interventions with Problems

If the problem is Miguel's position, then changing the position might decrease Joan's pain, but we can't expect an instant cure. Also, we know that there can be more than one problem simultaneously. If Joan's nipples are also infected, an antibiotic might be indicated. A woman can have sore nipples from faulty positioning and from *Candida* (thrush/yeast) at the same time. A woman can have sore nipples from faulty positioning and eczema or poison ivy at the same time. At this juncture, changing the position is the only solution that we can reconcile with the problem.

> Joan said that she might be willing to try again if she could stop when it hurt too much and if Mari would "get off my back about it." When we asked her to clarify what she meant, she said that she wanted Mari to promise that if she tried again right then that Mari wouldn't ever nag her again about stopping breastfeeding. Mari agreed, albeit reluctantly.

The hard foam pillow Joan was using situated Miguel too high compared with Joan's nipple. Also, the habit of lying Miguel on his back to nurse seemed to be connected with the pillow. Joan brought the pillow (a present from Mari) to the hospital and used it at every nursing.

> We removed the pillow, and turned Miguel "tummy to tummy" with Joan. A little throw cushion wedged under

> *Miguel's body took his weight but didn't change his opti-*
> *mal relationship to the breast. When Miguel's body was*
> *in the optimal position and his nose was opposite from*
> *the nipple, Joan could wait for Miguel to gape with a*
> *wide open mouth and come onto the breast with the*
> *nipple correctly placed for minimal trauma.[2] When Miguel*
> *was positioned optimally, Joan rated her pain as two on*
> *the five-point scale, down from the previous level of five.*

We know that Joan's nipple had considerable damage. Although it has happened, it's rare for a mother with painful, sore nipples to move from five to one on the pain scale in one nursing. Joan had been wary about even trying to nurse one more time, now that the pain was reduced, would she consider nursing another day?

8 Level 8—Evaluate Solutions and Interventions

The change in position moved Joan from five to two on the pain scale. She says it's still a little "uncomfortable." This could be from the residual damage to her nipple, or because more adjustment is needed. One way we'll be able to assess this is by observing the shape of her nipple at the end of the nursing. If the nipple is distorted, more adjustment will be needed.

We want Joan to know that pain is the best signal that Miguel isn't positioned optimally and that she should break suction and try again until she's nursing without pain. We also want to reinforce the idea that she should seek help for breastfeeding problems, not grit her teeth and bear the pain.

> *Joan nursed Miguel on her right breast for about 10 min-*
> *utes before Miguel released the nipple himself. We observed*
> *3–4 minute stretches of 2:1 and 3:1 suck to swallow ratios*
> *with 6:1 and 8:1 in between. Although a fissure was evi-*
> *dent where the scab had been, Joan's nipple was not dis-*
> *torted by this nursing. [Color Plate 4-2]*
>
> *We asked Joan if she would position Miguel by herself on*
> *the left breast, so that she could ask questions and get*
> *clarification from us if she needed any help. Joan was*

---

[2] A complete description of our positioning techniques can be found in *Maternal and Infant Assessment for Breastfeeding and Human Lactation.*

*picture perfect as she positioned Miguel and nursed on
her left breast.*

*We weren't surprised to see tears flowing freely down
Joan's cheeks. "I can't believe it doesn't hurt anymore."*

By providing her with solutions for the problem rather than the symptom, we helped Joan to have a pleasurable experience nursing Miguel if she chooses to do so.

Kate & Peggy

A different case of sore nipples with a different problem further illuminates the relationship between symptom and problem.

We received a call from Kate, the mother of three-week-old Peggy. Kate had painful, sore nipples since Peggy was three or four days old. She told us that her nipples hurt so much that she had to bite down on a receiving blanket for the first minute or two of nursing, then the pain let up, or she got used to it. She had tried almost every piece of advice anyone had given her. She came in to see us the morning after the call.

*Kate held the sleeping Peggy on her lap as she told us
about her breastfeeding history. She had nursed her two
older children now four and seven. She never had sore
nipples—just one case of mastitis. She nursed the older
children a year each and planned to nurse Kate for the
same length of time. "It's so weird, I would think my nipples were good and tough by this time. Someone told me
that I probably have a yeast infection, but the doctor said
no because Peggy doesn't have thrush or a diaper rash."*

 Level 3—Symptoms

(Same for this case as the one that precedes it.)

• Painful, sore nipples

The symptom is the same in this case, however the history is different. The onset of pain happened near in time to the onset of an abundant supply of milk. But formulating the problem requires more assessment information.

*Peggy started showing feeding cues and Kate got ready
to nurse. We observed areas near her nipple pores where
chunks of nipple were missing. Kate told us that first an
area would turn white then after a day or so it would
peel off.*

*We asked Kate to nurse Peggy in as close to the same way
she would nurse at home. She positioned Peggy in a
"tummy to tummy" position, Peggy took the nipple with
her mouth open at a 90-degree angle. Kate cringed and told
us the pain was almost unbearable. Peggy was sucking at
a suck to swallow rate of 12:1 with a chewing or piston
motion of the lower jaw. After about a minute, Peggy tipped
her head back, widened her mouth to about 120 degrees
and began swallowing rapidly in a suck–pause–swallow
pattern. Kate said, "It stopped hurting just then." The
change in pain coincided with Peggy's change in head position and her mouth opening.*

The problem in this case is with the latch process. Peggy has developed the habit of starting the nursing with a tight mouth and chewing
motion and then, after settling in, changing to a wider mouth, head
extended position. That the onset of this problem coincided with the
change from colostrum to abundant milk around the fourth day is not
a surprise. Peggy was born at 37 weeks gestation and may have been
overwhelmed by the volume of her mother's milk. An experienced
nurser, Kate already has a conditioned milk-ejection reflex. Peggy may
have learned to begin the nursing with a tight mouth to control the
flow, then, as she develops confidence that she can manage the flow,
she relaxes and opens her mouth wider. The initial tightness means
that the nipple does not go back far enough in Peggy's mouth for the
first minute or two of every feeding, so over time the nipple has
become damaged.

Even though Kate and Joan have the same symptom, painful,
sore nipples, the formulation for Kate at Level 4—Problem is that
Peggy's mouth opening is 90 degrees to start the feeding, changing to
120 degrees after one minute.

When we work on Level 5—Reconcile the history, assessment,
symptoms, and problems we become more assured that the problem
is correct. The solution and plan (Level 6) for Kate and Peggy is therefore unique and directed: Peggy should be encouraged to go to the
breast only with her mouth at 120 degrees or wider. This may take a
few days for Peggy to do consistently, but Kate should not allow

herself to be injured further. Peggy should open her mouth wide before Kate brings her to the breast. Level 7 is the level at which we reconcile our plan with what we determined to be the problem. We feel confident that opening Peggy's mouth seems to be an initial solution to the problem of the narrow angle of the latch.

> *We encouraged Kate to practice eliciting a wide gape with Peggy before repositioning her on the other side. Peggy cooperates and, after a few tries, Kate is able to achieve a pain-free latch. Kate needs to continue to be vigilant in order to be sure that Peggy doesn't close her mouth as her mother brings her onto the breast.*

Level 8—Evaluate Solutions and Interventions

Kate was able to nurse without pain on the second breast. When we called the next day she told us that Peggy was learning and when it hurt to latch she was breaking suction quickly and re-latching to avoid more damage to her nipples. Three days later her nipples were almost fully healed.

Anne & Carl

A third sore nipples case illustrates the same symptom with a different problem. Anne arrived at the Tuesday morning Nursing Mothers' meeting with two-week-old Carl. She told the other mothers and us that she was loving breastfeeding even though she still had painful, sore nipples. Anne told the group that she had come to the meeting in order to get some tips about what to do for her sore nipples. Anne was looking for a solution to her symptom not looking for a solution to the problem underlying the symptom.

> *As we observed Anne nurse Carl, we noted Carl gulping and pulling away from the nipple. His arms flailed and his legs kicked. As he pulled his head back, milk shot out into the room. Carl took a ragged breath or two and dove back onto the breast, sucking a few times and then letting go, breathing again and throwing himself back to the nipple. By this time, the nipple of Anne's right breast was shaped into a white wedge. Milk continued to spurt in between suckles.*

It was obvious to us that Anne and Carl had a style of nursing consistent with a mega supply of milk, a problem often called "oversupply." Oversupply is characterized by a volume of milk greater than the baby's current need, sore nipples (the baby's attempt to control the flow by crushing the nipple), much greater than expected growth, and a high volume of stools. Many babies whose mothers' have oversupply are fussy, especially after feedings. They may spit up large volumes of milk and want to nurse again. Anne had the symptom of sore nipples. We next need to assess Carl's growth pattern.

> *We asked Anne about Carl's weight and his weight gain pattern. Carl was born at 39 weeks gestation. He weighed 8 pounds 2 ounces when he was born and 7 pounds 11 ounces when he left the hospital 12 days before this group meeting. The day after leaving the hospital Carl weighed 7 pounds 12 ounces at the pediatric clinic.*

In the early newborn period an average weight gain of ½ ounce to 1 ounce per day is expected. If Carl gained an average of ½ ounce per day for 11 days, he should weigh about 8 pounds 1 ounce on day 14. If Carl gained an average of 1 ounce per day for 11 days he should weigh about 8 pounds 7 ounces on day 14. So we would expect Carl to weigh somewhere between 8 pounds 1 ounce and 8 pounds 7 ounces.

> *Anne stripped Carl and weighed him on the digital scale the mothers use in the Center. Carl weighed 8 pounds 14 ounces! We asked Anne about Carl's stools. "He poops about every time I feed him. Here's the diaper I just took off." Carl's diaper was completely covered with a thick coating of yellow seedy stool. Anne told us that Carl has 12–14 wet diapers, most with stool, every day.*

We proposed that we formulate Anne and Carl's problem as oversupply (Level 4). Can we, reconcile the history, assessment, symptoms and the problem we are proposing (Level 5)? Oversupply characteristics include greater than expected weight gain. (Carl has gained 17 ounces in 11 days, an average of 1½ ounces a day.) Anne reports that Carl has 12–14 wet diapers a day, most with significant amounts of stool as well. This is consistent with oversupply. Carl's behavior at the breast, the wedged nipple shape, and Anne's painful, sore nipples are also consistent with oversupply when the other components are present. Carl is fussy, according to Anne, but doesn't spit up much.

Level 6 is where we suggest solutions and plans for interventions. Anne believes that she has the problem of sore nipples not the problem of oversupply. We first need to explain our ideas to Anne and have her determine whether or not she agrees with our formulation of the problem.

> *As we describe the problem of oversupply with Anne, she agrees with our description of the problem. According to Anne, her partner Steve says that nursing Carl looks like "baby torture." He struggles and gasps and pulls away. His arms and legs flail around. "He just doesn't look like other babies do when they are nursing." It turns out that this is one of the reasons that Anne came to the group. She wanted to see what other babies look like when they nurse. She tells us that she's relieved to know that this isn't only about sore nipples. "I felt it was selfish to stop nursing because of sore nipples, but Carl didn't seem to be enjoying nursing either. One of the reasons I came today was to try to figure out what is normal."*

Because Anne had already been thinking about her situation, she was more open to solving the problem of oversupply. Not every mother is aware of her baby's behavior as he or she tries to cope with oversupply.

> *We explained to Anne that the solution for oversupply involves decreasing the volume of milk available for the baby. Two of the approaches we suggested were interesting to Anne. One was reducing the supply carefully by applying compression on the breasts in order to give the milk-making cells the message to make less milk. This could be accomplished by offering only one breast per feeding and removing milk from the other breast only minimally for comfort. The other was to remove milk on a regular basis and either store it or donate it to a milk bank. Eventually, if she wanted to, she could cut back on her supply by pumping less and less. We discussed the options with Anne. She thought the idea of donating to a milk bank was intriguing. She liked the idea that her abundant milk supply could help another baby.*

Level 7—Reconcile Prioritized Solutions and Planned Interventions with Problems

Either solution that Anne liked—reducing the supply or donating to a milk bank—will help to deal with the problem of oversupply.

Level 8—Evaluate Solutions and Interventions

Anne found that the solution that worked for her was to pump before nursing Carl. She began the process of becoming a milk bank donor. If decreasing the volume of milk hadn't changed the nursing pattern, we would have referred Carl to a tertiary center for a complete feeding study. The problem could have been a physical anomaly not a breast-feeding problem. Because Carl was able to handle a decreased flow of milk and suck–swallow–breathe in a regular pattern, a referral was not indicated at this point.

Jessie & Craig

Occasionally women have sore nipples well beyond the newborn period. The next case involves a woman who continued to have sore nipples at two months postpartum.

Jessie, a first-time mother living in a northwestern state, had been trying to solve the symptom of sore nipples for two months without success. When she saw our hostess' invitation for mothers with complex breastfeeding problems to be volunteers at our advanced issues in lactation consulting training program posted on the board in her pediatrician's office, she called our hostess to volunteer. Jessie arrived on Tuesday morning with two-month-old Craig.

> *"I've tried every remedy for my sore nipples and nothing has helped," she told us. "The pain has been excruciating." Jessie went on to list all of the remedies she had tried, including eliminating sugar and white flour from her diet. "For a while I thought I had a yeast infection in my breast. The shooting pains, the pain after the nursing, all seemed like yeast." Jessie was well read on the ways to solve sore nipple problems, had been buying yeast eliminating remedies at her health food store, and using a common yeast remedy that she painted on her nipples. "Nothing has helped though. Even the prescription drug for yeast that my physician prescribed for me didn't work. I took it for two weeks."*
>
> *We asked her about when the pain began. She told us that she remembered it happening in the hospital. "I remember coming out of the shower and it hit me. The*

*worst possible pain! It was in my nipples, shooting up
into my breast."*

*Craig was snuggled on Jessie's lap while we talked. He
moved his head back and looked straight up at his
mother. She stroked his head and he turned toward her
hand, rooting. She asked if we minded if she nursed
Craig and, of course, we didn't.*

*As she readied herself and Craig to breastfeed, we noted
her everted nipple, prominent Montgomery's glands, and
conical breasts. Craig lunged toward her exposed breast
with a wide-open mouth and began nursing. Within
moments he was nursing in a pattern of suck to swallow
that was 1:1 and 2:1. He had a few stretches of 8:1 but
continued a good rocker motion. Jessie told us that at
this point her pain was about 3 on our 1 to 5 scale. "You
wait," she warned us, "when he lets go it'll be 15!"*

So far, there is nothing in Jessie and Craig's history or the assessment
that helps us in formulating the problem.

*As soon as Craig released the nipple, Jessie told us that
the pain was starting. Her nipple was glowing com-
pletely white. Within moments it turned raspberry pink.
[Color Plate 4-3] [Color Plate 4-4] [Color Plate 4-5]*

Jessie's nipple color change is consistent with the problem of nipple
vasospasm or Raynaud's phenomenon of the nipple.[3]

Unfortunately there is no sure cure for Raynaud's although some
treatments have been helpful, such as the use of the prescription drug
Nefedipine.[4,5] Although seemingly rare, Raynaud's has been described
in published case studies, and we have seen several cases over the
years, probably because we are the "last stop" for so many mothers. In
some of the cases, such as Jessie's, there were no symptoms prior to
breastfeeding. In others, the mother tells us that her nipples have
turned white (or blue) and been painful when wet or exposed to cold

[3] Lawlor-Smith LS, Lawlor-Smith CL. Raynaud's phenomenon of the nipple: A preventable cause of breastfeeding failure. *Med J, Aust.* 166:448; 1996.

[4] Lawlor-Smith LS, Lawlor-Smith CL. Vasospasm of the nipple: A manifestation of
Raynaud's phenomenon; case reports. *Br Med J.* 314:644; 1997.

[5] Lawrence RA, Lawrence RM. *Breastfeeding: A Guide for the Medical Profession.* St.
Louis, MO: Mosby, Inc.; 1999.

as far back as she can remember. One mother told us that beginning at 14 or so she had to stop swimming because the nipple pain was so great under her cold, wet bathing suit. Sometimes the mothers also have a history of Raynaud's in their fingers and/or toes. Some have no personal history but have parents with the symptoms. One mother had no prior Raynaud's symptoms, no family history, but had infected nipples and had been hospitalized for mastitis prior to the onset of the painful nipples of Raynaud's.

Rachel & Sarah

> *Rachel called the warmline one Tuesday morning in July. "I was going to ask if I could come in and see you about my sore nipples, but Sarah is so miserable. I think she must be teething. She doesn't have a fever or anything; she's just crabby. I don't know if we'll make it." We assured Rachel that she could drop in anytime before five. "Maybe if she falls asleep I'll try to put her down in the car seat." Rachel sounded doubtful but did come in to the Center that afternoon.*

 Level 1—History

Rachel and Sarah had been nursing happily for four and a half months when suddenly Rachel had sore nipples. Sarah has gained well, sleeps well, and has been a pretty happy baby until the last few days.

> *"My mother thinks I should wean her, that she's getting spoiled. Maybe I haven't been spending enough time with her and she's crabby because of that." Rachel went on to tell us that since school got out she had a constant parade of visitors. "You know what it's like to live on Cape Cod," she laughed, "people say they are coming to see you and the baby, but actually spend their time at the beach." She told us that so far this summer, her brother and his family and her sister and her family had spent vacations at her house. Her mother had been staying with her for weeks. "She lives in Florida, so it's nice to see her, and she wanted to be with my brother and sister and their families too."*

Level 2—Assessment

We don't have much of an assessment so far.

 Level 3—Symptoms

- Painful, sore nipples
- Newly crabby four-month-old

 Level 4—Problem Formulation

We really don't have enough of an assessment to even begin formulating a problem list.

> *Sarah begins to stir and Rachel immediately coos to her and unfastens the car seat. When she lifts Sarah out she begins to cry in earnest. When she opens her mouth we can see a white carpet on her tongue. Using a gloved finger we check the insides of her cheeks. Her cheeks are coated too. When we assess Rachel's breasts there is a shininess that may indicate* Candida *(yeast or thrush). [Color Plate 4-6]*

We can now formulate a problem.

- Possible *Candida* (yeast or thrush) affecting both Rachel and Sarah

Level 5—Reconcile the History, Assessment, Symptoms, and Problem

The problem of *Candida* reconciles well with the history (sudden onset), the physical assessment of the white carpet coating in Sarah's mouth, and the glossy coating on Rachel's breast.

 Level 6—Generate and Prioritize Solutions and Plans for Intervention

> *We proposed our formulation of the problem and proposed intervention to Rachel: a visit to Sarah's health care provider for a diagnosis and prescription. Rachel called her pediatric office from her cell phone. The pediatric nurse practitioner could see them right away.*

Level 7—Reconcile Prioritized Solutions and Planned Interventions with Problems

The problem of *Candida* is best managed by prescription medications. A referral to the appropriate prescriber is the protocol for *Candida* at the Center.

Level 8—Evaluate Solutions and Interventions

> *Rachel called the next morning. The nurse practitioner had prescribed medication for* Candida *and instructed Rachel to think about possible vectors for transmission of the fungus (e.g., pacifiers, toys, etc.). Rachel was cleaning Sarah's toys and the breast pump parts.*

These cases illustrate the importance of seeking the root cause or causes of the problem encountered rather than just treating the symptoms.

Further Reading

Lawlor-Smith LS, Lawlor-Smith CL. Raynaud's phenomenon of the nipple: A preventable cause of breastfeeding failure. *Med J Aust.* 166:448; 1996.

Lawlor-Smith LS, Lawlor-Smith CL. Vasospasm of the nipple: A manifestation of Raynaud's phenomenon; case reports. *Br Med J.* 314:644; 1997.

Lawrence RA, Lawrence RM. *Breastfeeding: A Guide for the Medical Profession.* St. Louis, MO: Mosby, Inc.; 1999.

Discussion Questions

1. Have you ever been in the position of our hostess Mari who seems to be more invested in breastfeeding than her sister? What was that like for you? How have differing views about breastfeeding affected your relationship with a friend or relative in the long term?

2. What is a *vector*? How is a vector related to transmission of thrush? Make a list of possible vectors that you might want to give to a mother who has the problem of *Candida*.

Chapter 5

Reconciling Problems

"An undefined problem has an infinite number of solutions."

—Robert A. Humphrey

This chapter addresses the consulting dilemma we call numerators in search of denominators:[1] In this situation there are multiple, often confusing symptoms, and the one piece of information—the key—that anchors the symptoms to a problem may be missing or difficult to discern. Although cases of numerators in search of denominators are rare, they are illustrative of the complexities of lactation consulting.

Kim, Dan, & Max

We traveled to a rural community hospital to teach a five-day training program. We were met at the airport by one of the hospital nurses, Elaine, on the afternoon before the program was scheduled to begin. Elaine was excited about the training, telling us that they were going

---

[1] This term has been used in discussions of medical problem-solving. It may have been originated by: Spodick DH. Revascularization of the heart—numerators in search of denominators. *Am Heart J*. 81:149–57; 1971.

to start a nurse-run, 24-hour breastfeeding help line. We chatted informally about the kinds of questions we get on our three-county warmline at the Center for Breastfeeding and how difficult it is to be assured of the accuracy of an over-the-phone assessment.

We think of our warmline as an outreach to the community, with many of the calls being referred to a health care provider, USDA's Special Supplemental Nutrition Program for Women, Infants and Children (WIC), and the Visiting Nurses. According to our logs, almost all of the mothers are encouraged to be seen in person either by us or by their health care provider. We told Elaine that we use protocols, just as the hospital does. We also use maxims such as "flu in a nursing mother is mastitis until proven otherwise," because we have found that new mothers suddenly feel ill but don't necessarily have symptoms that would lead them to even examine their breasts for redness or lumps. We ask mothers who are ill to check their breasts using a mirror and call their physician or midwife.

Elaine went to work the evening shift at the hospital after dropping us off at our hotel. She called us just after 8 P.M. "You won't believe what happened! Do you remember how you said that flu in a nursing mother is mastitis until proven otherwise? Well, right after I got to the hospital, a nurse, Kim, who is home on maternity leave called to ask if she could breastfeed even though she's coming down with the flu. I told her to check her breasts and she couldn't find any red areas or lumps. She had a temperature of 103°F, so they were bringing her into the Emergency Department."

At 9:30, Elaine called back to tell us that they had admitted Kim. Because they had a room with two beds free, the baby and Kim's partner, Dan, were staying overnight. The baby, Max, is only four days old and exclusively breastfeeding. They cultured everything they could think of and started Kim on a broad-spectrum IV antibiotic until the results of the cultures came back and a more specific antibiotic could be prescribed. There was no redness on Kim's breast and Elaine couldn't find any lumps either. The only breastfeeding problem was sore nipples. Kim had been complaining about sore nipples almost from the first nursing. Max was a great nurser according to the staff and the birth was idyllic according to the hospital's standards.

By the next morning, Kim was no better. She was getting fever-reducing medications, but her temperature was still 103°–104°F. The staff, many of whom were Kim's friends, dropped in during their off hours to help Kim nurse Max. Kim became progressively more ill as the day went on.

Elaine asked us to visit Kim after class, around 5 P.M., and we were able to do so. Dan told us that Kim was complaining of pain when she breastfed. He was worried that nursing was taking too much out of Kim. Dan was appropriately concerned. He wondered if we could teach him how to help Kim nurse lying down. "She's so out of it, but she wants to keep breastfeeding. When she sits up she's dizzy. If I could position Max while she's lying down it would really help."

 ## Level 1—History

Kim gave birth to Max five days before without complications. On the afternoon of day 4 at home, Kim developed a high fever of unknown origin. Her temperature ranged between 103–104 degrees and was not effectively reduced by fever-reducing medication. She is hospitalized and is receiving IV antibiotics. Max and Dan are rooming-in with Kim. Kim is dizzy when she sits up to nurse.

 ## Level 2—Assessment

Kim's breasts have been examined for mastitis twice and there are no lumps or redness. She has complained of nipple pain while nursing since the first day. According to Dan, she is unable to nurse Max sitting up because of dizziness.

 ## Level 3—Symptoms

- Fever of unknown origin
- Nipple pain while breastfeeding
- Dizziness affecting ability to nurse sitting up

 ## Level 4—Problem Formulation

Kim has an underlying problem that has not been diagnosed. The fever is a symptom of this problem. The dizziness may be due to the fever or part of this underlying problem. At this point we have insufficient information about the nipple pain symptom to formulate a related problem.

The one piece that we can help with is the problem of Kim needing to nurse lying down because of her dizziness when nursing sitting up.

⑤ Level 5—Reconcile the History, Assessment, Symptoms, and Problems

At this point, we can reconcile the problem of Kim needing help nursing lying down with the history, assessment, and symptoms. We acknowledge that this is only a small part of a larger picture.

⑥ Level 6—Generate and Prioritize Solutions and Plans for Interventions

We can teach Dan how to position Max so Kim can nurse lying down. We may be able to assess Max's nursing during the teaching session.

> *We chatted informally with Dan and Elaine about the hallmarks of a good position while watching Max for feeding cues. As Max began stirring, Dan helped Kim to lie on her right side. Elaine placed a pillow at her back for support. When her hospital gown was lifted, the two lower quadrants of Kim's right breast were observed. The skin was bright red having an almost burned appearance. Elaine checked under the left breast and the two lower quadrants were also bright red. No redness was visible when the breasts were positioned against Kim's chest as in sitting or standing.*

This finding of bilateral redness is a medical emergency. Streptococcal infection has been associated with bilateral appearance of mastitis.[2] The finding is consistent with the history, assessment, and symptoms. Once the true nature of Kim's problem was discovered, effective drug treatment was initiated. She recovered rapidly, and was discharged with a comfortably nursing baby within a few days.

This case illustrates how even when there are multiple symptoms, the one piece of information that anchors the symptoms to a problem may still be missing. This is what we call numerators in search of denominators, and we teach our students to make a list of all of the possible symptoms (numerators) and look for the problem or problems that will explain as many symptoms as possible (denominators).

---

[2] Schreiner RL, et al. Possible breast milk transmission of group B streptococcal infection. *J Pediatr.* 91:159; 1977.

Donella & Cody

This is another case of numerators in search of a common denominator.

> *We received a warmline call from Donella, the mother of an 18-week-old baby boy, Cody. She was concerned because Cody was "acting weird" and she wanted to give him prune juice. She had talked the idea over with her neighbor who told her that she always gave her kids prune juice. Donella remembers her mom giving her younger siblings prune juice, too. We asked Donella about feeding Cody. She said that he was mostly breastfed. "But Cody is constipated and it's really bad, and my friend told me this was normal for breastfed babies." In our conversation with Donella, we found that Cody had stooled at least once a day until a week or so ago. The stools were yellow and seedy or brown and clay-like. "He usually used to go a little every time I nursed or one big potty once a day or so. But the last big one was seven days ago. He had a little potty in his diaper once this week, but that's it. He is sort of crying and sad. A little crabby, no, a lot crabby. I feel as though a good purge is what he needs."*

 Level 1—History

Donella is describing a change in mostly breastfed 18-week-old Cody's behavior that is troubling her. He had a change in his previously regular bowel habits and disposition.

 Level 2—Assessment

It is impossible to assess Cody over the telephone. We can assess Donella's emotional state as agitated and concerned. We know that Cody has had a significant change in his stooling pattern, and, during the same time period, developed an increasingly irritable disposition.

 Level 3—Symptoms

- Change in bowel habits (for which mother believes prune juice is indicated)
- Irritability

Level 4—Problem Formulation

Although prolonged periods of time without stooling are widely reported as normal in breastfed babies, prolonged constipation can also be a symptom of a medical problem. We don't have enough assessed information to determine a problem, although we know that the pediatrician should be consulted about the constipation/prune juice issue. Therefore we need to continue with the assessment.

> *"Have you noticed any change in Cody's appetite or in his interest in nursing?" we asked. Donella told us "Yes, Cody usually loves to nurse first thing in the morning, but this morning he wasn't crabby anymore, he just whimpered at my breast. He acts like he can't even hold up his head."*

We can add this new information to our assessment. Cody has had a change in appetite and his mother has noticed weakened head control.

Level 3—Symptoms

- Change in bowel habits for seven days
- Irritability at first, now whimpering
- Poor appetite (a change)
- Weak head control (a change)

Our list of symptoms has increased. Clearly, we cannot formulate this into a breastfeeding problem. The symptoms are consistent, however, with the problem of infant botulism, a medical emergency. According to the Centers for Disease Control (CDC), botulism should be suspected in an infant under a year old with symptoms including constipation, lethargy, poor feeding, weak cry, bulbar palsies, and failure to thrive.[3] Progressive weakness, impaired respiration, and sometimes death might follow these symptoms. A laboratory test of stool is available but the results may not come in for more than a week.

Level 4—Problem Formulation

The symptoms are not consistent with a breastfeeding problem, but potentially with the medical emergency infant botulism.

- Potential medical emergency

---

[3] Centers for Disease Control. Infant botulism—New York City, 2001–2002. *Morbidity & Mortality Weekly Report*. 52(02):21–24; Jan. 17, 2003.

Level 5—Reconcile the History, Assessment, Symptoms, and Problems

As we review the information that we have obtained there is nothing that would reassure us that this is a benign situation or a breastfeeding problem.

Level 6—Generate and Prioritize Solutions and Plans for Interventions

The plan we developed is that Cody should be transported to a medical facility as soon as possible. We tell Donella that we are very concerned about Cody and believe he should be taken to the emergency department right away. She tells us that her neighbor is with her and can take them to the hospital without delay. Donella will call the doctor's office from her neighbor's cell phone as they drive to the hospital.

Level 7—Reconcile Prioritized Solutions and Planned Interventions with Problems

If we believe the problem is a medical emergency, the solution is appropriate. Of course, we have only talked to Donella over the telephone, but we are impressed with the gravity of the symptoms she is describing.

We know that infant botulism, although much more common and deadly in formula-fed infants, has been reported in breastfed infants.[4] Infant botulism results from the germination of swallowed spores of botulinum toxin that, according to the CDC, produce clostridium that colonize in the large intestine temporarily. The annual incidence of infant botulism in the United States is two cases per 100,000 live births.

Level 8—Evaluate Solutions and Interventions

Donella called us from the hospital pay phone. "Thank you, thank you. They told me that coming here was the right thing to do." On arrival in the emergency department Cody's temperature was 105°, and because of respiratory weakness and upper-airway obstruction, mechanical ventilation was initiated. We asked Donella if she needed a breast pump in order to keep up her milk supply for Cody

---

[4] Arnon SS, Damus K, Thompson B, Midura TF, Chin J. Protective role of human milk against sudden death from infant botulism. *J Pediatr*. 100(4):568; 1982.

until he's ready to nurse again. She told us that she never pumped but she wanted to. "I want to hold him in my arms and nurse again. I want him to smile up at me. He loves nursing." Donella cried into the phone. We made arrangements to meet her with a pump and teach her how to use it.

Donella pumped conscientiously during Cody's hospitalization. Cody was kept on mechanical ventilation for 14 days. Botulinum toxin type B was identified 8 days after admission in stool samples. Cody was discharged after 26 days and recovered fully.

Cases with numerators in search of denominators are often the most complex.

Heidi & Forrest

A nurse, Janet, who had attended a one-day workshop in a large metropolis, called one morning. "I'm very concerned about my daughter Gina's friend, Heidi, and her baby, Forrest, who is 20 days old. The baby is gaining very slowly. Heidi is married to a very famous man and lives in a protected world. They are very private, but I'm afraid that they are putting the baby at risk."

Janet works in a public prenatal clinic. "I don't know enough to help her, but listening to my daughter I just know that Heidi needs help." We asked if Heidi was taking Forrest to a pediatrician. She told us that she was, but she wasn't taking their advice about breastfeeding. "If she called you, would you talk to her?" We agreed to talk to Heidi in order to give her the name and contact information of a skilled lactation care provider in her area who we felt could be trusted with Heidi and her family's privacy. We were going to the same metropolis in a week, maybe we could meet Janet for dinner.

Heidi called the next day. We offered to give her the name of a local contact but she wanted to tell us what was going on first. Forrest was born vaginally after a 20-hour labor. Forrest weighed 7 pounds 6 ounces. "I had a doula, that was great, but I was so tired afterward I just slept and slept. Forrest would wake up and nibble at my nipple but he didn't really latch on."

Heidi continued with her story. On day 4 she expected her milk to "come in" but it didn't so she started pumping with the lightweight portable pump she bought on the Internet while she was pregnant. She couldn't pump more than a coating on the bottom of the bottle. She felt pumping was a waste of time since Forrest now would latch on and nurse for 40 minutes an hour—every hour. "He just sucked and sucked so I knew he wasn't getting much, and when I pumped I got so little."

At the first pediatric visit the doctor was concerned that Forrest was still at discharge weight (6 pounds 14 ounces) at 8 days. "They wanted to start formula so I thought, I'm not coming back here." She found a store in the telephone book that sold breast pumps [and also got 15 minutes of breastfeeding advice]. Heidi went to buy a pump. They agreed that she shouldn't feed the baby formula and sold her another breast pump that was ordinarily a rental pump. "When I got that pump I thought my problems were solved, but I still couldn't get much milk and Forrest still nursed all the time."

So I got the name of a lactation center and went there for a consult. They watched us nurse, told me that the latch was fine and sold me on a hospital grade pump. I thought, wow how dumb am I? I have three pumps now and not enough milk for one!" At this point Forrest was 16 days old.

Heidi had been told that her pump was the problem twice. Obviously the thought process of the people whose advice she had sought had been to think of the symptom as not enough milk and the problem as the wrong pump. Listening to Heidi's story, we were thinking that the symptom was poor weight gain and inadequate milk supply and/or delivery and that the problem was as yet unknown.

"I knew I had to take Forrest back to the doctor, but not the first one. I simply didn't want to hear that I should give him formula." This point of view had been reinforced at both the pump store and the lactation center. Heidi called her doula for a recommendation of a pediatric office that wouldn't tell her to use formula. The doula gave a suggestion and Heidi went when Forrest was 20 days old for a checkup. The weight check indicated that Forrest was 7 pounds 2 ounces, not yet up to birth weight. The pediatric nurse practitioner suggested that formula be delivered with an at-breast feeder. Heidi told us that she was really angry at the suggestion. The nurse practitioner wanted Forrest to get at least 20 ounces of formula or

*breast milk or a combination of the two every day. The
practitioner told Heidi that she would get enjoyment out
of feeding him at her breast and Forrest would get the
nourishment he needed. Heidi was indignant. "I'm not
going back there either." She did purchase the at-breast
feeder, however, but she had not used it.*

The pediatric nurse practitioner saw the symptom configuration the
same as we did—as poor weight gain and inadequate supply or delivery of milk. However, she went right to a solution—feed the baby and
preserve the breastfeeding experience—without a more in-depth check
of history, assessment, or symptoms.

Heidi was not convinced. This is often the case when the problem
is not formulated and articulated to the mother, it's more difficult to
engage her in the solution. What we often find then is a lack of com-
pliance with the proposed solution. That's what Heidi is expressing.
Heidi has the means to "just go to someone else." Other mothers just
drop out of the helping network. So far we haven't a clue as to what
Heidi and Forrest's problem is but we agree with the pediatric nurse
practitioner that this is a baby that needs to be fed. We wonder if the
nurse practitioner had prescribed donor breast milk if that would have
been more palatable to Heidi.

*We are wondering about Heidi's history. Has she ever
had breast surgery? ("No.") Had anyone asked her
before? ("No.") What do her breasts look like? ("Similar
to each other. Normal looking nipples.") Did she have
changes in pregnancy? ("Yes, I can see blue veins.")*

*What about Forrest? According to Heidi, the pediatric
nurse practitioner found no problems with him except
his poor weight gain.*

Breastfeeding is a performance activity. We have Heidi's report that
the person she consulted at the lactation center found no problems
with the nursing. We wonder if they compared before and after
weights. Had Forrest transferred milk? If so, why wasn't he gaining?
Many women have problems collecting milk when pumping, even if
they have babies who are gaining right along.

*We asked Heidi about her vaginal flow or lochia, espe-
cially any change in her vaginal discharge in terms of
color and quantity. We asked about her discharge since
Forrest was born. She told us that it had always been*

*red, sometimes it was light enough for a panty liner, but
usually she needed 4–6 pads a day. Was it still red today
(day 25)? "Yes."*

Given our new information we might reconstruct the levels as follows.

 Level 1—History

The mother has had 25 days of serous lochia. The baby has been gaining poorly, and on day 20 (the last weight check) was not up to birth weight. Pumping produces only very small amounts of milk with a variety of pumps.

 Level 2—Assessment

We have no assessment.

 Level 3—Symptoms

- Poor weight gain of the baby
- Small amounts of milk pumped with a variety of pumps
- Continuing bloody discharge to 25 days

 Level 4—Problem Formulation

The only problem that fits with this grouping of symptoms and history is retained placental fragments.[5] These cases have been previously described. The theory is that the retained placental fragments may be capable of secreting sufficient progesterone and other hormones of pregnancy to keep the mother from moving from pregnancy (in which colostrum is produced) to abundant amounts of mature milk usually by three days postpartum.

 Level 5—Reconcile History, Assessment, Symptoms, and Problems

We feel that we can meet the reconciliation requirements of Level 5 as described in the research presentation by Anderson.[5]

---

[5] Anderson AM. Disruption of lactogenesis by retained placental fragments. *J Hum Lact*. 17(2):142; 2001.

⁶ Level 6—Generate and Prioritize Solutions and Plans for Intervention

Heidi should be seen by her midwife or obstetrician as soon as possible. Ultrasound examination of the uterus, for example, may determine if there are fragments. Removal of any fragments that have been found is done by the surgical procedure commonly called D&C (dilatation and curettage) or D&E (dilatation and evacuation). Without prompt evaluation, Heidi could hemmorhage.

We didn't hear from Janet for several days. She called to make dinner plans for Saturday night when we would be in her town. On Saturday, Forrest would be 29 days old. We wondered how Heidi and Forrest were doing. "Gina is talking to Heidi about whether you could visit her on Saturday before we have dinner. Would that be okay with you?" We agreed and tucked information about the local lactation care provider into the ticket case to give to Heidi when we saw her.

There was a note from Janet at the hotel detailing our pickup information. We had consulted on high-profile cases before so were familiar with the process. We were not to bring cameras or cell phones, tape recorders, or anything else that could be construed as an invasion of privacy. We shouldn't take notes or be prepared to have them confiscated.

We had no idea what we might or might not need. Would we just meet Heidi and give her the phone number of the contact? Was Heidi expecting us to consult on her case? What was going on with them now? What did Heidi's physician or midwife find? We had no idea, so we had had a pharmacy drop off a digital scale with breast-milk-intake function at the hotel. We had a small bag from the Center packed with small pieces of equipment we might need for our assessment or tools for an intervention. Our plan was to leave everything in the car and retrieve it only if needed.

We were expected at the security gate and the guard let us, along with Gina and Janet, go up to the house. We stood outside until the security people in the house invited us in. We were escorted into a dramatic room with spectacular views and offered coffee and tea. Heidi bounded into the room smiling and holding a thin almost one-month old Forrest. "My super, super baby!

We finally did it, we have MILK!" We exchanged introductions, hugs, and air kisses as Heidi exuberantly told her story

"They found fragments! I wasn't due for my postpartum check for another week. I called my midwife right after talking to you. She sent me for an ultrasound right away. They did the D&C that afternoon and removed the fragments that they saw on the ultrasound. Within hours I had milk!"

Just then Heidi started to nurse Forrest. She positioned him at her left breast and swiped her nipple across his mouth. He opened his mouth grasped around the nipple and began to suckle. After 30 seconds of an 8:1 suck to swallow ratio, Forrest settled into 1:1 and 2:1 for about 3 minutes. He returned to 8:1 and then to 1:1 and 2:1. Heidi was ebullient. "He's getting something, I just know it." We asked if this was the way Forrest had always nursed. She told us that this was new. Suddenly, at around 2:00 that afternoon, after the D&C, my breasts started feeling full and leaking milk. Forrest is thrilled, he's been nursing up a storm."

 ## Level 2—Assessment

By observation the baby is suckling with a rocker motion and periods of 1:1 and 2:1. Gulping and swallowing are heard. Milk is seen dripping from the unsuckled breast. We used the scale we brought and found that Forrest transferred 2.8 ounces on the second breast.

 ## Level 3—Symptoms

Reviewing the previous symptom list, we can now eliminate a few items.

- Poor weight gain
- ~~Small amounts of milk pumped with a variety of pumps (inadequate production?)~~
- ~~Continued bloody discharge at 25 days~~

 ## Level 4—Problem Formulation

Forrest needs to catch up the weight he didn't gain. He needs pediatric supervision in the long term.

(5) Level 5—Reconcile the History, Assessment, Symptoms, and Problems

Although one potential reason for Forrest's poor gain has been postulated, there could be additional problems, therefore ongoing supervision is important. Heidi's past behavior indicates that she might reject advice she doesn't agree with.

(6) Level 6—Generate and Prioritize Solutions and Plans for Interventions

Solutions and interventions include test-weighing Forrest before and after multiple feedings to assure Heidi (and us) that he is indeed being nourished. Find a pediatric practice whose advice Heidi will follow.

(7) Level 7—Reconcile Prioritized Solutions and Planned Interventions with Problems

We need to reconcile the solution with the problem because we are concerned about Forrest's weight gain. Heidi agrees.

(8) Level 8—Evaluate Solutions and Interventions

> *Janet called a few days after we returned home to tell us that Heidi and Forrest returned to the pediatric nurse practitioner who had suggested the "at breast" feeder for a weight check. Forrest had gained and was now 3 ounces above birth weight.*

Everyone whom Heidi consulted had an opportunity to look for the denominator but they never asked the question that would get to the key numerator or symptom. Lactation care providers should encourage mothers with prolonged, red, vaginal discharge to seek professional assessment.

Maggie & Dakota

Here's another case of numerators in search of denominators.

> *Maggie called on the recommendation of her lactation consultant from a town about 80 miles away. She wondered if she and her 13-month-old baby, Dakota, could*

*come and see us about her sore nipples. Even though
Dakota wasn't nursing anymore (he had weaned 2 weeks
before, but she was hopeful he might nurse again), the
nipples hadn't responded to any treatment she and the
lactation consultant had tried and now it was even
worse. She could come the next day. She would not use
any new products until she saw us.*

One of the reasons that we are happy to take a second, or even tenth
look, is that as time passes, things change. We have seen women who
may have had a positioning problem and yeast be treated for *Candida*
and still have sore nipples. They look and look for new yeast treatments when what they need is a position tune-up. We have also found
women who think that they have a resistant strain of yeast who actually have sore nipples because of a new pregnancy.

Yeast can be found in combination with strep, staph, eczema, and
poison ivy.[7] We have also seen "yeast" that was actually a dermatolog-
ical reaction to a nipple care product.

*Maggie and Dakota arrived the next day. After such a
long ride, Dakota couldn't wait to be put onto the floor.
He cruised around, exploring, as his mother had some
tea and visited the bathroom. She sat on the couch and
told us about her yeasty nipples. "It's not just my nipples,
it's my areola and up onto my breast." She showed us
her breasts. The skin was excoriated over a large area of
the breast and areola with a few places where deep
crevices of skin were missing. There was no mistaking
the smell of yeast, however.*

*How about Dakota? He had no rash on his bottom or
white patches in his mouth that we could see. We asked
her about pain. "Yes, it's painful. That's probably why
Dakota weaned. He knew it was hurting me. If I could
take care of this problem, maybe he would start again."
We asked her about vaginal yeast problems and she told
us that she had horrible vaginal yeast but was using
over-the-counter preparations. They were not working
and her perineum was in as much pain as her breasts.*

*The lactation consultant she had seen previously had
recommended that Maggie go to her physician to get a
prescription for a systemic yeast infection. Maggie refused.
"I just didn't want anything going through my milk that*

---

[7] Powers N. Burning pain is not always yeast. *ABM News and Views.* 6(2); 2000.

*could hurt my baby," she said hugging Dakota. "I'm into
natural things, so there was no way I would take a drug
while breastfeeding. I'll just put up with it if you can't
think of anything else for me to do."*

Let's take a look at where we are at this point.

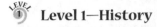

Level 1—History

Maggie gave birth 13 months ago to her third child, a full-term
baby boy, Dakota. She had sore nipples from the start. Dakota
weaned two weeks ago. Maggie believes that his weaning is connected to her pain. Dakota has never had a diaper rash or white
patches in his mouth according to his mother. In the past few
months, the skin on her breast, areola, and nipple has become excoriated, reddened, and cracked. Numerous antifungal skin preparations have been used without success. Maggie did not seek medical
treatment because she did not want to expose her nursing baby to
medications via her milk.

Level 2—Assessement

The skin of Maggie's breast and areola appear red and excoriated. A
yeasty odor is noted. Maggie tells us that she also has the same problem in her vagina and perineum.

Level 3—Symptoms

- Painful breasts and nipples (pain also reported in the perineum)
- Skin lesions
- Yeasty odor

Level 4—Problem Formulation

There is not enough information to determine the problem.

Level 5—Reconcile the History, Assessment, Symptoms, and Problems

There is nothing that we know from the history, assessment, or
symptoms, beyond the yeasty odor, that helps us to determine the
problem.

Level 6—Generate and Prioritize Solutions and Plans for Interventions

The plan we presented to Maggie was to have a thorough examination from her primary care provider, including blood tests and perhaps a referral to a dermatologist.

Level 7—Reconcile Prioritized Solutions and Planned Interventions with Problems

Since we are unable to formulate a breastfeeding problem, a medical consult is needed.

Level 8—Evaluate Solutions and Interventions

We asked Maggie to keep in touch with us because we had never seen a case like this before. She agreed.

> *The next month, Maggie called. Her physician had pre-scribed a systemic antifungal medication. "It's working, but only a little. The doctor says I'll have to go to a der-matologist." Maggie said that she would call us again if she learned anything new. Almost six months later, Maggie called again to tell us that blood tests showed that she was HIV positive. She was devastated. Crying, she explained that she hadn't known that Dakota's father was HIV positive. She had been monogamous and thought she was low risk for any sexually trans-mitted disease. "The doctor became suspicious when the yeast infection didn't clear up. He thought it might be a problem with my immune system . . . and it was," she sobbed.*

Maggie reported that her sons had all been tested for HIV, and all had been found to be uninfected, including Dakota. "Thank God my babies have been spared," she exclaimed. Maggie told us she had separated from her husband and moved back home with her parents. She was taking antiretroviral treatments, and was responding well and feeling stronger.

She told us that her family and community was rallying around her. "I'm hoping to have many more healthy years with my boys," she shared, "but I'm putting my house in order."

In this case, like the others in this chapter, the symptoms are compelling and beyond what would be expected with a simple breastfeeding problem. In the case of Elaine, the symptoms of "flu" were actually symptoms of a medical emergency, a serious strep infection; in the case of Cody, the symptoms of constipation and poor feeding were due to botulism; Heidi's milk "came in" after removing retained placental fragments, and Maggie's yeast infection was due to her HIV status. These cases illustrate the importance of being open to uncommon or unusual problems.

Further Reading

World Health Organization, Department of Child and Adolescent Health and Development. *Mastitis: Causes and Management*. Geneva: WHO; 2000.

The Academy of Breastfeeding Medicine. *Clinical Protocol Number 4—Mastitis*. Available at: www.bfmed.org.

Arnon SS, Damus K, Midura TF, Chin J. Protective role of human milk against sudden death from infant botulism. *Journal of Pediatrics*. 100:558; 1982.

Anderson AM. Disruption of lactogenesis by retained placental fragments. *J Hum Lact*. 17(2)142; 2001.

Discussion Questions

1. A case of infant botulism is presented in this chapter. What are the symptoms of food-borne botulism in adults? How is it contracted? What is the relationship of infant botulism to Sudden Infant Death Syndrome (SIDS)?

2. One of the cases in this chapter dealt with the problem of retained placental fragments in a breastfeeding mother. What key question would have revealed the symptoms of retained placental fragments at earlier breastfeeding consultations? When do breastfeeding mothers start to menstruate after giving birth?

Chapter 6

Outgrowing Solutions

Besides learning to see, there is another
act to be learned—not to see what is not.

—MARIA MITCHELL, ASTRONOMER, EDUCATOR
(1818–1889)

This chapter explores situations where the mother and baby may be experiencing problems because they have outgrown a solution for an earlier problem. Sometimes the old solution may be causing new problems.

Fiona & Raphael

On a rainy spring day, we met Fiona and her adorable four-month-old baby Raphael.

> *Fiona had called for a consult appointment. When she arrived we were working with another mother on positioning. We found her a comfortable chair within the same room, and asked her to fill out a self-administered history form while we finished up with the other mother and baby. Fiona made herself comfortable, placing Raphael on the floor for some "tummy time," and filled out the form, while*

obviously listening in on, and eventually entering into, the discussion with the other mother.

Our physical setup encourages this type of interaction. The Center's consult room is a large living room space with numerous rockers, rotating rattan chairs, and couches. Privacy can be achieved, if a mother wishes, by rotating chairs, using screens, or moving to a small, private consult room, but we find that mothers rarely choose these options. The companionship of other mothers and babies and the parallel learning opportunities seem only to enrich mothers' experiences and understanding of their own situations.

> *When the other mother left, we asked Fiona what brought her to the Center. She told us that breastfeeding was very important to her, "I really believe in it, you know. It is the best thing for babies. But I find I'm getting to the end of my rope." When asked to tell us what was making breastfeeding unbearable she replied, "The schedule, the mindlessness of it, it's all too much. Lots of my friends are nursing and they seem to be able to get out of the house and hang out together, but I'm so busy at home I can't get there. I feel like I hardly have a life. Don't get me wrong, I love being Raphael's mother, but some days I just feel like a feeding trough." Her face flushed with feeling (embarrassment? anger?) as she spoke.*
>
> *"Tell us about a typical day," we requested. She then recounted the events of the previous day, including 10 breastfeedings, ten 20-minute pumping sessions, 2 loads of wash (hung on the line and later collected and folded), a 1-hour nap for mother, two 1-hour naps for baby, and 5 hours of sleep at night.*
>
> *"Wow, that's a busy day," we responded. "Tell us about the pumping. Are you planning to return to work?"*
>
> *"I'm a graduate student," she said, "I'm on leave for this semester. When I do return in the fall, I'll be able to bring him to Boston with me. My mom lives a few miles from campus and she'll watch him. He'll be eight months by then."*
>
> *"What is your reason for pumping now?"*

"Because he's a preemie. The nurses told me I had to pump after every feeding for 20 minutes or so to stimulate my milk production."

Further questioning identified that Raphael had been born at 34 weeks gestation, weighing 5 pounds 2 ounces. He was in the neonatal intensive care unit for 3 days for stabilization, and then was transferred to the nursery for 3 weeks. He was fed only Fiona's pumped milk, plus some added minerals. His growth was satisfactory, maintaining fetal growth rate after the first week of life.

"Looking over the form you filled in, we don't see any history of problems for Raphael."

"No—he's an angel. I just wish he'd sleep a bit more, but otherwise he's been very healthy."

 ## Level 1—History

History provides few clues other than prematurity and maternal concern with "doing the right thing." The pregnancy and birth appears to have been uncomplicated, other than by premature birth. Maternal and infant history appear otherwise unremarkable.

 ## Level 2—Assessment

Raphael began to roll around on the floor, apparently trying to locate his mother. We asked her to strip him down and weigh him on our breast-milk-intake scale. He weighed 16 pounds 2 ounces and measured 25⅝ inches, plotting out at the 75th percentile for both weight and length. His weight-to-length ratio was between the 50th and 75th percentiles.

> *She then changed his diaper, carefully washing her hands afterward, and got a small plastic case out of her diaper bag. She lowered her head and said, "I'm embarrassed to show you that I use a nipple shield. I know that they are not popular with breastfeeding people. My friends are all really into nursing. They can't believe that I'm still using the shield. They tell me to just chuck it."*
>
> *"Well, popularity aside, can you tell us why you use it?"*

"The specialist in the Neonatal Intensive Care Unit (NICU) said there was a new study out that said premies feed better with a shield. They take more milk, and suckle better," she said, a bit defensively.

"Oh yes, we're familiar with that study,"[1] we replied, "very interesting findings. Have you been using the shield since he was in the NICU?"

"Yes. Anything that keeps him growing is OK with me. The specialist wouldn't have recommended it if she didn't think it was necessary," she replied.

"Would you consider trying this feeding without the shield?" we asked.

"Why? Don't you think it's a good thing for me to use?"

"It may have been helpful for Raphael in the beginning. But, it may not be necessary at this point. In fact, it may lower the amount of nipple stimulation your brain perceives, which could have an effect on your milk supply."

"I don't have any problems in that area," she chuckled. "I've got enough milk in my freezer, my mother's freezer, and my neighbor's freezer to feed 10 babies."

"Sounds like you do," we said. "We'd like to talk about that, too, but Raphael looks interested in some food. Let's see what he thinks about nursing on a bare breast."

When she offered her breast to Raphael without the shield, he looked a bit surprised, but latched on happily. "Look at that," she marveled, "he doesn't seem to miss the shield at all." He moved through a period of 10:1 sucks, reaching 2:1 or 1:1 sucking in less than a minute. He detached from the breast about 4 minutes later. We asked Fiona to put him back on the scale after she burped him. He had transferred 4.1 ounces in 4 minutes, according to the scale. Fiona was right—no problem with milk production or transfer here!

Fiona then offered him the other breast, which he took right away, nursing nutritively for most of 5 minutes,

---

[1] Meier PP, Brown LP, Hurst NM, Spatz DL, Engstrom JL, Borucki LC, Krouse AM. Nipple shields for preterm infants: Effect on milk transfer and duration of breastfeeding. *J Hum Lact.* 16(2):129–31; 2000.

then falling sleeping off the breast, and rolling his eyes with a glorious "milk-drunk" expression. We didn't disturb him for a second weight. Fiona denied any feeding-related pain or physical discomfort for herself or the baby.

Level 3—Symptoms

- Difficulty completing an overwhelming workload related to pumping and feeding
- Disconnection from friends related to workload and embarrassment about shield use

Level 4—Problem Formulation

- Breastfeeding is too much work and has caused some embarrassment

Level 5—Reconcile the History, Assessment, Symptoms, and Problems

- All appear to reconcile

Level 6—Generate and Prioritize Solutions and Plans for Interventions

- Simplify breastfeeding routines to provide more time for Fiona to reconnect with her pre-Raphael self and her circle of friends
- Reduce and eventually remove pumping schedule
- Remove shield
- Encourage outings and support activities

Level 7—Reconcile Prioritized Solutions and Planned Interventions with Problems

- Plan seems to account for all problems identified

Level 8—Evaluate Solutions and Interventions

Fiona was impressed with the amount of milk Raphael transferred without the shield. She seemed cautiously relieved that the shield might no longer be necessary. She was also very interested in the scale, and in how it calculated the amount of milk transferred by multiplying the change in weight by the specific gravity of milk to calculate ounces transferred. She told us that she was studying mathematics in graduate school.

"Going back to the idea of pumping," we asked, "would you be willing to step down that schedule somewhat?"

"Maybe," she replied. "You don't think it's necessary?"

"Not unless you do intend to provide milk for 10 babies," we replied. "Have you considered becoming a milk bank donor?"

She expressed interest in this concept, and said she would look into it. "It would simplify life, though, if I didn't have to pump after every feeding, and clean the darn thing after every pumping."

We agreed. "What a lot of work you've been doing. You are working so hard to do the right thing. We commend you for all that hard work. Sounds like you're ready to reap some of the benefits of breastfeeding for your lifestyle. What do you miss most about your life before Raphael?"

"Don't even get me started! Having coffee with my friends, discussing the latest novel, going to see the latest independent film, roaming the stacks in the library to see what's new . . . so many things," she reminisced.

"You mentioned that you have a large circle of friends with babies. Would it be possible for you to get together with them?"

"Well, now that I don't have to pump after every feeding, maybe I could! I've been avoiding some of them because they are very judgmental about the shield thing, but maybe I don't need that any longer. Wow!" she finished. "Maybe I could run by Starbucks on my way home. They're probably there right now."

We helped her pack up and transfer Raphael to his car seat. She agreed to call us the next day to follow up on the shield. We encouraged her to drop the number of pumping sessions slowly, so that breast fullness could be minimized.

She called us the next day to happily report that she had tossed her shields in the trash. "What a relief!" she said. "I feel more like myself already. I had a great time at Starbucks, everyone was so happy to see Raphael and me. We're going to start a stroller walking/book club."

Further follow-up contacts with Fiona found that she had reduced pumping sessions to once daily. She sounded stronger and more sure of herself at every contact.

Through connection with her friends, and shedding the unnecessary burdens she had perpetuated, she came to find much more enjoyment and fulfillment in her new life with Raphael.

Sarah & Isaac

Less than three months later, we met Sarah, a woman with a similar problem related to practices that were once beneficial, but were no longer helpful.

Sarah's son Isaac was born at 32 weeks' gestation. He was hospitalized for 6 weeks. Sarah diligently pumped to provide most of his nutrient needs during the hospitalization. After discharge, she exclusively breastfed Isaac, and she also continued to pump 8–10 times daily. Her own mother was unable to produce a full milk supply for her, and she was not going to let that happen to Isaac.

She was referred to the Center at 12 weeks' postpartum for help dealing with recurrent bouts of mastitis. When asked the reason for seeking help, she replied, "I want to nurse Isaac for at least one year. I'm planning to spend this year at home, fully focusing on him. But I'm getting run down by these constant infections and his tummy troubles. I need help."

 Level 1—History

Sarah is a primipara whose history includes gestational diabetes, preterm labor, three bouts of mastitis, and two bouts of candidiasis.

Isaac was born at 32 weeks' gestation and had been exclusively breastfed since hospital discharge.

Level 2—Assessment

Isaac slept deeply through the interview, so we were not able to assess a feeding. Review of Isaac's immunization record shows that his current weight is in the 75th percentile for his corrected age, with his length at the 20th percentile. Weight/length ratio is slightly above the 95th percentile.

> *When asked about her comfort, Sarah told us that she feels no pain associated with feedings, but does report that her baby has feeding-related discomfort. "Poor little thing," she elaborated, "he sputters and chokes at the breast. He has massive poops, usually overflowing his diaper right down to his socks and way up to his neck. He passes gas all the time."*
>
> *She reported that she nurses Isaac every time she sees feeding cues (totaling 12 feedings yesterday). Because she has heard that the high-fat milk comes at the end of the feeding, she has made a habit of keeping him on the first breast for a minimum of 10 minutes, then burping him and putting him back on the other breast for a minimum of 10 minutes. When asked how he responds to this, she replied, "he gets really mad when the milk lets down on the second side. He tries to pull off, but I can get him to stay by pressing against my breasts like this (she demonstrates pressing her fingers into her breast in a scissor-like clamping fashion)."*
>
> *When asked what she thought was causing the problem, she stated that she thought the baby's symptoms to be a reaction to an unidentified food in her diet. She said she was consuming a very restricted diet of rice, a few fruits, and boiled chicken. "Nothing I do seems to make any difference. I'm practically starving, and he's still having a reaction."*

Level 3—Symptoms

- Sarah: Recurrent mastitis and candidiasis

- Isaac: Explosive, abundant bowel movements; sputtering and choking at the breast; and gastric discomfort after feedings. These symptoms have not responded to maternal dietary manipulation.

Level 4—Problem Formulation

- Overabundant milk supply causing symptomology for both mother and baby

 ## Level 5—Reconcile the History, Assessment, Symptoms, and Problems

A few other possibilities surface as we reconcile these levels: undiagnosed neurologic or gastrointestinal problem or developmental delay in baby; unresolved or partially resolved breast infection; or inflammation due to reabsorbed milk produced in response to frequent nursing and pumping.

Level 6—Generate and Prioritize Solutions and Plans for Interventions

- Work to decrease milk supply by
  - Practice baby-led feeding. Reinforce satiety cues. Offer one breast until baby shows satiety cues. When satiety cues are seen, remove baby from breast; offer the other breast. If baby refuses, stop feeding.
  - Decrease pumping by dropping one scheduled pumping session per day. Begin to shorten the length of time spent pumping.
- Observe breasts daily for any red, inflamed areas.
- Observe baby for changes in gastric discomfort, stooling, etc.

Level 7—Reconcile Prioritized Solutions and Planned Interventions with Problems

Solutions address the possible problem of oversupply. Add referral to pediatrician to rule out other pediatric problems. Add referral to OB/GYN to rule out other maternal problems.

Level 8—Evaluate Solutions and Interventions

When presented with these possible solutions, Sarah responded with concern. "How will I know he is getting enough milk if I limit him to one side and stop pumping?" We discussed the self-regulating ability of the older baby, and talked about ways of assessing his intake by looking for satiety cues, counting soiled diapers, and getting periodic weight checks at his pediatric clinic.

Sarah seemed a bit uncertain about our suggestions, but said she was willing to try them for a few days. We worked out a follow-up plan. As she began to gather her things together to leave, Isaac awoke, stretched, looked around and filled his diaper with audible force. Laughing, we welcomed Sarah to change him and stay for a feeding so we could observe his reaction to suggested changes. She agreed. By the time she was ready to feed him, her shirt was soaked with milk let down from both breasts. As she brought him to the breast, her well-tuned ejection reflex had his face quite damp. He complained a bit about this, but eagerly attached to the nipple. His suck to swallow rhythm began at 2:1 and within about a minute he was gasping and sputtering through another powerful let down. We encouraged her to take him off the breast and hand express some of the flow to slow the feeding down a bit. He reattached after resting for about a minute. During this time, he had another audible bowel movement. After two additional minutes of 3:1 to 1:1 suck to swallow nursing, he removed himself from the breast. "How could he possibly have gotten enough in that short a feeding?" she asked us. "Look at him closely. He knows how full he is . . . he is the only one who knows," we replied. Together we listed the satiety cues that were visible: relaxed body posture visible from his opened hands to his curled toes; half-closed eyes; goofy facial expressions ranging from drunken to a clown-like frown; relaxed lips.

Sarah moved Isaac to her shoulder when he began to squirm a bit. Soon he produced an audible belch, and relaxed onto her shoulder. "Should I give him the other side now?" she asked anxiously. "Let's wait until we see some feeding cues," we replied. We sat and chatted for 10 minutes, watching him for signs of hunger. "Nope," she finally said, "he's out cold. OK, I'm going to take him home and see how this works."

Sarah called us later that week to say that she had just come home from Isaac's pediatric visit.

"The doctor was very happy with his growth. He read your report, and agrees that we should just wait and see if he feels better after a week or so on this new plan. He is less gassy, that's for sure, but he's still pooping a lot."

When asked about her breast comfort, Sarah replied that she was down to four daily pumping sessions lasting five minutes or so. "I'm removing as much milk now as I was before, but I'm doing it much less often, so I guess my supply must be decreasing."

One month later we checked in with Sarah who was attending a support group meeting.

She reported that Isaac was almost never gassy anymore, that feedings were much shorter and easier, and that she was down to pumping only once a day "for a relief bottle for the freezer." She pronounced herself proud to be mastitis-free for a whole month. She had a new problem, though; Isaac was now teething and trying to chomp on her nipple at the beginning of feedings.

And so it goes for many moms . . . one problem solved, another one on its way. Time for another consult!

Juliana & The Triplets

We received a call on the county warmline from Juliana, a breastfeeding mother of triplets.

"How can we help you today?" we asked.

"Do you remember me, Juliana from the Island? I have three breastfeeding triplets."

"How could we forget that? How are you doing?"

"Nursing is going just fine. They are such fine healthy boys. They're getting teeth, but I haven't been bitten yet," she replied wryly. "What's bothering me now is that the boys won't stay in their blankets in the crib."

"Hmmm . . . remind us . . . how old they are now?"

"Six months. They just won't stay swaddled anymore."

"Tell us why you want to swaddle them."

"In the NICU, the nurse told me that they would stay asleep longer and be more comfortable if she swaddled them tightly and lay them together in the crib so they could sense each other's presence. I still try to soothe them this way, but they won't stay wrapped up. They crawl on top of each other and get in all kinds of mischief. I just don't understand why they won't lie down and go to sleep."

Level 1—History

Growing, apparently healthy triplets. Mother has had no problem maintaining a full milk supply.

Level 2—Assessment

Telephone consult—no visual assessment. Feeding recall and reported weights sound fine. Reported difficult behavior appears appropriate for developmental stage.

Level 3—Symptoms

- Irritation with baby behavior

Level 4—Problem Formulation

- Outdated expectations?

Level 5—Reconcile the History, Assessment, Symptoms, and Problems

- Appear to be reconciled

Level 6—Generate and Prioritize Solutions and Plans for Interventions

- Offer support and developmental information

Level 7—Reconcile Prioritized Solutions and Planned Interventions with Problems

- Appear reconciled

Level 8—Evaluate Solutions and Interventions

> *We talked for a while about the changing developmental needs of babies. Juliana mentioned that she was feeling very lonely and disconnected. She was staying at home all day with her babies, because she was concerned about them becoming ill. We talked to her about the broad range of support activities available in her community, and encouraged her take part in some of the group activities. Perhaps a nature walk with the babies in their stroller would allow her to be with others in a relatively germ-free environment? We also referred her to her pediatric nurse practitioner for a recommendation on how much she needed to protect her babies from interaction with others (another outdated practice for her six-month-old babies?).*

Thoughts

New parents are extremely observant of the way their babies are cared for by health care professionals. Parents absorb and do their best to duplicate the infant-handling techniques, mannerisms, and beliefs of those they deem to be authorities. One of the challenges of working with parents is helping them to see and examine the appropriateness of these absorbed characteristics. We can help parents find their own expertise by reflecting on what has worked, what is working, and what is no longer working for them.

Further Reading

Kavanaugh K, Meier P, Zimmermann B, Mead L. The rewards outweigh the efforts: Breastfeeding outcomes for mothers of preterm infants. *J Hum Lact.* 13(1):15–21; 1995.

Nyqvist KH. Breast-feeding in preterm twins: Development of feeding behavior and milk intake during hospital stay and related caregiving practices. *J Pediatr Nurs.* 17(4):246–56; 2002.

Discussion Questions

1. Have you worked with other mothers like Fiona who are struggling with adapting their interactions with their baby's developmental needs? How did you identify this problem? What type of interactions might have helped Fiona to adapt more gradually to Raphael's changing needs? How might the support needs of mothers of premature or sick infants be different from those of full-term, healthy infants?

2. What might be the underlying causes of recurrent mastitis? How would you recommend dealing with these causes?

3. What strategies would you offer Sarah for dealing with Isaac's teething discomfort? What are the possible benefits and risks of any strategies proposed?

Chapter 7

Missing Pieces

*A problem well stated is a
problem half-solved.*

—RICHARD BUCKMINSTER FULLER, PHILOSOPHER,
ARCHITECT (1895–1983)

In this chapter we explore the problem of discarding information or failing to examine information because it seems uninteresting, unimportant, or irrelevant. Either the mother or the care provider may believe that a question is not worth asking, or the consultant has information that is not considered in the formulation of problems.

Siobhan, Kevin, & Aisling

Telephone counseling is challenging because of the lack of visual cues to the nature of the problem, and the difficulty reading emotional content of speech. Late one night a call came in on a home phone line from an old college friend, Siobhan, who had just had her first baby. She and her husband Kevin live on the West Coast.

"Hi! I'm calling to tell you that I had a baby girl 5 days ago."

"Oh! How wonderful! How was the birth?"

"It was long and arduous, but we made it through. It got scary after birth, though. Aisling stopped breathing and turned blue about an hour after delivery, while I was trying to nurse her."

"How terrifying! What did you do?"

"I yelled for help. Kevin took Aisling and checked her vital signs, tilting her head back to open her airway. By the time the nurse arrived she was breathing again. They said it was too short a time to have caused any brain damage, but they put her on a monitor and kept her on it for another day. There were no other episodes, so they told us it was just a fluke."

"How are you doing with that now?"

"OK, I think. I keep her right near me and keep checking on her breathing, but I guess that's pretty normal."

"Absolutely, especially after a scare like you had. And how is it going with feeding her?"

"It took her a while to get started. She was pretty groggy after the scare. It was hard to nurse her with the monitor, but we figured it out. She's been pretty sleepy since we brought her home, which is why I'm calling you. Kevin has been trying to wake her up to nurse, but she's really out of it."

"Hmmm . . . why don't you put him on the phone, if he's right there."

"Actually, he can get on the extension. Can you pick up, Kevin? OK, he's on now."

Kevin and Siobhan are both physicians. We hope to tap into their clinical skills to elucidate the situation.

"Congratulations, Kevin! How is life with baby going?"

"It's been a wonderful, wild ride! I know Siobhan told you about the anoxic event. Now that we're back home, and ready to get our life together off to a great start, we

can't wake the kid up. I've done two complete neurological work ups on her, and she won't budge."

"You probably remember that newborns have different sleep cycles than adults. Deep sleep is really difficult to disturb, but she should cycle into light sleep within 30 minutes or so, and then she should be more easily wakeable."

"What should we do until then?" Siobhan asked.

"Strip her down to her diaper, and lay her skin-to-skin on your chest, under your nightie. Keep her there until you see REM sleep, little wiggly body movements, or any mouthing or vocalizing. Then move her closer to the breast."

"Take her out of the blanket?" Siobhan asked worriedly. "Won't she get too cold?"

"Your body will warm her perfectly. You can leave her hat on if you wish, but take everything else off but the diaper."

"OK, I'll give it a try," Siobhan answered sounding uncertain. "Gosh, she's adorable. I wish you could see her. She has short, caramel-colored hair, with a little curl to it . . . and the most heavenly blue eyes you can imagine. And her skin is the most gorgeous shade of apricot you can imagine—like a Tuscan sunset."

This description raised red flags for us. Kevin and Siobhan were red-haired, white-skinned Irish descendants.

"She sounds so beautiful," we answered. "Can you tell me more about her skin tone? Has it always been apricot-colored?"

"No, she was very pale the first two days," Kevin responded. "Oh my gosh, you're right. She's jaundiced. Holy cow! How did I miss that? What should we do? Take her in for a work up?"

"A certain degree of hyperbilirubinemia is expected in the newborn, as you know, but [that] could certainly be influencing her alertness and her drive to feed."

"Yep, I see it all now. As soon as we're done, I'm going to call her pediatrician. He owes me a favor, so I feel OK

*about getting him out of bed for some new-parent jit-
ters," Kevin asserted.*

"What else should we do?" Siobhan asked.

*"Keep her skin-to-skin, in the restaurant, as we say, so
she can get right to the food when she wakes up. When
she is at the breast, squeeze a little milk right into her
mouth to keep her interested. Start hand expressing or
pumping after every feeding, and in between feedings if
she isn't nursing 8 times or more in 24 hours. And call
back anytime, keep us posted!"*

*Kevin called the next afternoon to say that Aisling had
been readmitted to the hospital for phototherapy. Her
bilirubin level was markedly elevated. Siobhan was
pumping her milk every 2 hours and it was being gavage
fed to Aisling. They were waiting on lab results. If the levels were falling, they would allow the baby to be fed at
breast, wrapped in a fiber-optic blanket, and returned to
the lights. Kevin reported that Siobhan was feeling bad
that they had missed the jaundice, but that she was coping well with the rehospitalization.*

*"This whole experience has taught me so much about
breastfeeding," he confessed. "I used to think it must be
easy, no big deal. Boy, did I have a lot to learn!"*

Missing the information of jaundice made Aisling's problem appear to
be a breastfeeding problem. In fact it was a physiologic problem—her
high bilirubin level was making her groggy. Once the nature of the
problem was identified and treated, breastfeeding improved. The
anoxic event, of course, increased the likelihood of jaundice.

Noel, Wayne, & Heather

During the morning coffee break of a 1-day hospital workshop, a staff
nurse, Gwen, asked if we would come up onto the floor at lunch and
take a look at a mother's nipples. The mother and baby had to be discharged by dinnertime when the baby would be 48 hours old. The
mother's nipples were flat and they had not had a single breastfeeding.
Gwen explained that the mother had not been able to breastfeed her
son, now 3, because of the same problem. The father has been giving

the baby formula in a bottle. The nurses just didn't want to let this mother leave without a chance at breastfeeding.

> *"We all feel so bad. We worked so hard with breastfeeding when she had her little boy 3 years ago and it didn't work. Now we feel as though we have another chance at breastfeeding, but we can't get this baby to nurse on these flat nipples either."*

> *We agreed to come up to see the mother during the lunch break. Gwen, who had talked to us that morning, as well as the staff lactation specialist, escorted us. After being introduced to the mother, Noel; Wayne, the baby's father, and Heather, the baby, we asked Noel to tell us what was happening. "It's just like the last time, my nipples are too flat. My babies don't want to nurse on such a flat nipple." Noel showed us her nipples. They were, indeed, flat.*

> *We asked Wayne to take the baby's clothes off (except for the hat and diaper) and to position her chest against Noel's chest with her head midway between Noel's breasts. A flannel blanket was put loosely over Heather and Noel to hold in the baby's body heat. In addition, we reassured the parents that Noel's breasts would adjust their temperature in order to keep Heather warm.*

This is a technique we often use to assess the baby's ability to orient to the breast. We have the baby positioned skin-to-skin while we talk to the adults. This gives the baby time to use the stepping–crawling reflex and move toward the breast. This is an assessment strategy that, we have found, often becomes an intervention.

> *We asked about how long her nipple had been flat and Noel told us that she first noticed in seventh-grade gym class that her nipples didn't stick out like the other girls'. "They do pucker up when we make love," she blushed. Wayne nodded. "The babies just don't get it. Even when I stuff my nipple in Heather's mouth she doesn't seem to know it's there. Neither did Sean."*

> *At this point Heather was lifting her head and bobbing. Her eyes were closed, her hands fisted, and her mouth was making sucking motions. We asked how Noel knew it was time to feed Heather and she and Wayne both told us that they were feeding "on demand." "When she cries*

we change her diaper and try to feed her. She gets to my breast and either fusses or goes to sleep. After a half-hour or so of trying to force her to take my nipple we give in and give her the bottle. That's what she's looking for." We asked why they wanted to breastfeed and they listed out several reasons, all related to the health of the baby. "I knew all these things when I had Sean. He never nursed, not even once. He's had ear infections and bronchitis. I just know that he should have been breastfed."

At this point, Heather was 2 inches away from the nipple and bobbing her head actively. We asked Noel and Wayne about the labor and birth. "It was fine. I had an epidural, so the labor didn't bother me much." Wayne added, "We went practically natural with Sean and I was begging for a cesarean at the end. I couldn't stand to see Noel in pain. So this time she agreed to an epidural."

As we prolonged the conversation by asking the details of the labor, Heather reached Noel's left nipple and began licking at the base. All eyes turned to Heather as she began the familiarization process.[1] Noel's nipple responded to Heather's mouthing behaviors by becoming progressively more everted. Within five minutes she gaped and began suckling. Wayne grabbed Noel's hand, leaned over and kissed her as they watched Heather nurse expertly. Minutes later, Noel repositioned Heather on her right breast using the cross-cradle hold. Heather latched on and nursed effectively. Each of Noel's nipples was everted momentarily at the end of the nursing.

As we review this case, there are two issues that stand out in our minds. One is the way a part of the assessment can become an intervention. In this case we wanted to observe the desire of the baby to approach the breast and the ability of the baby to self-attach. Heather had the desire to reach the breast and the ability to self-attach. Key factors included time, lack of constraint on Heather's head and shoulders, and the stepping-crawling reflex. It was a bonus that Noel's nipple responded by everting.

---

[1]The stepping–crawling reflex and baby's first attachment can be seen in the video *Dr. Lennart Righard's Delivery Self-Attachment.* It is distributed by Health Education Associates; 508-888-8044, fax 508-888-8050.

The second issue, and the theme of this chapter, is discarded information or aspects not considered. In this case Heather's newborn abilities to self-attach were not considered or evaluated by the staff in the shadow of the importance of Noel's flat nipples. Part of this was due to the nurses' memory of their shared feelings of failure with Sean; they discounted the baby and focused on the issue that was the same in both cases, Noel's nipple. No one had assessed Heather's self-attaching behavior at the breast, only Noel's positioning of Heather. Especially in the early days, the intact baby should evidence a desire to access the breast and the ability to self-attach. With babies who are nursing poorly, for example, we might assess a baby's ability to nurse in a variety of positions. As with this case, the assessment of a baby may become an intervention when we find that the baby nurses well in cross cradle but not in the "football" position or vice versa.

Let's look at the levels prior to our assessment.

Level 1—History

Noel attempted to nurse her older child Sean, who is now 3, but he never latched. The second baby, Heather, is now 44 hours old and has never latched. The mother's description of prior breastfeeding attempts included pushing her breast into Heather's mouth, and that Heather fussed or slept at the breast. The parents believe that the lack of success at breastfeeding is due to Noel's flat nipples. The nipples have been flat as long as Noel can remember, but both parents report that the nipples evert in response to sexual stimulation. Heather has been formula fed via a bottle since birth.

Level 2—Assessment

The mother, Noel, has two apparently flat nipples.

Level 3—Symptoms

- Flat nipples
- Baby fusses or sleeps at the breast

Level 4—Problem Formulation

Because we are unable to formulate a problem, we need to assess Heather's behavior at the breast, especially her desire and ability. If we believed that the flat nipples were a problem not a symptom, we would have focused our attention on the nipples. However, flat nipples are rarely a problem if the baby is able to configure the breast; then suckling can be successful.

We asked Wayne to place Heather in a skin-to-skin position and observed her stepping–crawling reflex and her familiarization activity at the breast. We can now add to our assessment.

Level 2—Assessment

The mother, Noel, has two flat nipples. Heather is able to approach the breast, self-attach, gape, and suckle effectively. At the end of the self-attached feeding, Noel's left nipple is everted. She nurses on the right breast in the cross-cradle position and everts that nipple as well.

Level 3—Symptoms

The symptoms have now changed.

- Flat nipples evert in response to suckling
- ~~Baby fusses or sleeps at the breast~~

We no longer have a problem to formulate in response to this symptom. Assessment by itself, appears to have been an intervention.

Kelly, Andy, & Sam

It's not natural to ask, "What information have I discarded?" In this next case, during a home visit, we see that the mother has discarded information.

Kelly was a mother who seemed full of energy and optimism. She breastfed her now 22-month-old son, Andy, for 15 months. At the time of weaning she was 4 months pregnant. She wanted to continue nursing throughout her pregnancy, and tandem nurse the two children, but had such excruciatingly painful nipples she had to stop. Her new baby is also a boy, Sam. Sam has been diagnosed as having Down Syndrome.

Kelly called us at 5 weeks postpartum for help. She told us that she had turned her energy toward making nursing work, but Sam had gained poorly. At first, the pediatrician advised her not to worry; babies with Down Syndrome often gain slowly, but now at 5 weeks, the pediatrician was concerned and had advised Kelly to call the Center for a feeding evaluation or to start formula.

Kelly wanted to breastfeed Sam, so she called the Center for help. She knew that some of the poor health outcomes associated with Down Syndrome (obesity, lowered IQ, Type I Diabetes) might be mitigated by breastfeeding. She had been pumping, she told us, but over the course of a day's pumping only collected an ounce or two. She was able to pump more in the early weeks.

Kelly found getting Andy and Sam out of the house to the Nursing Mothers' Group meeting or for a consult to be almost impossible. Could we make a home visit?

 ## Level 1—History

Prior breastfeeding experience of 15 months of 22-month-old, Andy. The new baby, Sam, has been diagnosed with Down Syndrome and at 5 weeks is still at discharge weight, 7 pounds 11 ounces. Kelly is able to pump only a few ounces a day, although she was able to pump more the first two weeks.

 ## Level 2—Assessment

We haven't seen Kelly or Sam.

 ## Level 3—Symptoms

- Poor weight gain at 5 weeks (still at discharge weight)
- Diagnosis of Down Syndrome
- Lowered amount of milk collection via pumping compared to early weeks

 ## Level 4—Problem Formulation

We will make a home visit to observe Kelly nursing Sam because Kelly is unable to get both children out of the house and come to the Center. Without a complete assessment, we are unable to formulate a problem.

Kelly's home is located down a long, dirt driveway, not unusual in our rural area. As we pull up in front of the house to park, we can hear at least one stereo, a TV, and a radio through the closed windows of the home. We ring the front doorbell for a minute or two before deciding to walk around the house to the kitchen door. A fenced in area contains four dogs that begin barking when we come around the house. Kelly is in the kitchen and opens the door when she hears the dogs. Andy is scooting around her feet on a mini plastic car, banging into her, and making ambulance siren noises. Every surface in the kitchen is covered with dishes.

Kelly thanks us for coming and explains, gesturing to the dishes, how she tries to get her siblings to help with the housework but they are very busy even now during summer vacation. She has three teenaged siblings, two brothers and a sister, who live in the house, along with her husband, Andy Senior. Her father, a fisherman, is gone most of the time so she is the parent. "I've been the parent ever since my mom died when I was 15. She died of lung cancer after a long illness. My youngest brother was 3 when she passed away. He's now 13. I'm the only mother these kids really remember, and with my dad away fishing so much, my husband, Andy, really is like a father to them." The dogs continue to bark.

At this point toddler Andy dashed out of the kitchen into the house and we followed Kelly and Andy into a family/ living room. The room was unoccupied although a large-screen TV was tuned to a sports channel playing at a high volume.

We noted that the stairs were covered in foam and duct tape. Andy ran up to the stair landing and threw his body over the stair rail. He landed on a sofa in the family room, seemingly strategically placed, jumped a few times and ran up the stairs again. We noticed that every corner in the room was protected with foam and duct tape. "Andy is so active," Kelly laughed, "we just decided to try and keep him from harm. The foam and duct tape are doing the trick." We wondered about Sam. He was upstairs with 14-year-old Caitlin. Kelly started up to get him. "Caitlin is so great with Sam. She never had any patience with Andy, but Sam is such a snuggle-bunny, Caitlin can't get enough of him."

It was now 11:30. We wondered about when it was that Sam had last nursed. Kelly thought for a minute and remembered nursing first thing in the morning, "It was about 7 or 7:30, when my husband was leaving."

> *Kelly returned with Sam who was well swaddled and sleeping. We asked her about pumping and she told us that she tries to pump, but she gets so little that it's almost not worth it. "I used to have so much milk with Andy that I pumped once a day or so if my breasts were full. My breasts are almost never full now, so it's not worth pumping."*
>
> *We asked Kelly how many times a day she nursed Sam. She told us that she didn't keep track because she was nursing "on-demand" as she had with Andy. She positioned Sam at her breast but Sam showed no signs of feeding readiness or interest in nursing. Kelly held Sam at her breast for a minute or two before Andy began climbing around on the kitchen table among the dishes. Kelly shouted at Andy a few times, telling him to get down. When he didn't, she put Sam down in a baby chair, and went into the kitchen to remove Andy from the table. Andy hopped onto the Big Wheel and began to race between the furniture, making ambulance siren noises again. Kelly picked up Sam and walked to the bottom of the stairs, screaming up to Caitlin.*

We are now able to begin to formulate the problem. We think that Kelly has intellectually grasped the diagnosis of Down Syndrome for Sam, but has not integrated the meaning of the diagnosis in her everyday life, and especially related to breastfeeding.

 Level 4—Problem Formulation

- *Inadequate number of feedings.* Sam is simply not able to "demand" at a sufficient decibel level to penetrate Kelly's awareness. This is partially due to the home environment, partially due to her prior experience nursing Andy, who was a very demanding nurser, and partially due to the typical characteristics of a baby with Down Syndrome.

- *Inadequate feedings.* Because of Sam's weak muscle tone and possibly caloric deprivation, he is unable to suckle effectively.

- *Low milk supply.* Because of infrequency of both feedings and pumpings there is a good chance that Kelly's milk supply is low. Her previous experience with nursing Andy did not prepare her for having to pay attention to her milk supply with Sam.

Level 5—Reconcile the History, Assessment, Symptoms, and Problems

The problems we formulated integrate well with the history, symptoms, and assessment.

Level 6—Generate and Prioritize Solutions and Plans for Interventions

The solutions and plans must address the problem of the inadequate nourishment of Sam. We need a frank conversation with Kelly about noticing and nursing Sam in the chaotic environment in which he lives. Sam is unable to signal to Kelly about his feeding needs in a way that penetrates her concentration. She will have to change the way she thinks about how a baby makes his needs known. She will also have to work to build up her milk supply. Like a baby with Down Syndrome, a pump does not have obvious feeding cues. Kelly will have to learn to watch the clock and pump and feed frequently.

We have every confidence that Kelly will be able to build up her milk supply, however, it will take regular pumping, 8-to-10 times a day. In addition, she will have to feed Sam, perhaps as many as 10-to-12 times a day. We can teach her how to observe his subtle hunger cues, how to awaken Sam, and how to maximize the feedings.

We will also recommend before and after feeding weights for a week or more as well as close pediatric follow-up. If she is able to pump any amount of milk, perhaps she can use an at-breast feeder until Sam is able to transfer milk well.

We discussed the problems and proposed interventions with Kelly, focusing on how she thought she could fit Sam's need to nurse more often and more effectively into her life. We also discussed pumping frequently, and regularly, not just when her breasts were too full. We discussed the use of an at-breast feeder, a scale with breast-milk-intake function and pediatric supervision. Kelly told us that she had a lot of milk in the freezer. During the first 3 weeks of nursing Sam, her breasts had been very full and she pumped just for comfort. She assumed, at that point, that everything was going well.

Level 7—Reconcile Prioritized Solutions and Planned Interventions with Problems

Kelly told us that she realized that she had let Sam and his needs blend into the noisy active family. Caitlin was happy to cuddle Sam, something that she had never been able to do with Andy. This further separated Sam from Kelly's awareness.

Level 8—Evaluate Solutions and Interventions

We defrosted 2 ounces of frozen milk from Kelly's freezer and showed her how to feed Sam through a tube at her breast. Sam was able to form a seal and, typical of babies with Down Syndrome, fell into a suck to swallow pattern around the milk flow.

By the next day, Kelly had pumped 10 ounces in 24 hours and was supplementing the freshly pumped milk with frozen milk. Sam had begun to suckle more actively. Kelly found that keeping Sam with her in a sling was one solution to the problem of him becoming lost in the large and noisy family.

This case is illustrative of the same issue as in Noel and Heather's case: An important piece of information had been discarded as irrelevant—the babies' abilities. In both cases the mothers had a prior experience that affected the way they thought about the current baby. Sean never nursed and it was assumed Heather wouldn't either. However, Heather was able to nurse once she was given the opportunity to self-attach; Sam was unable to make his needs known to his mother through the noise level of their home, and due to her memories of nursing Andy just a few months earlier. Nursing an active, demanding toddler is the polar opposite experience to nursing a newborn with Down Syndrome.

Adora & Bella

In this next case, we were asked to visit a hospital within driving distance. The nurses were having problems with a baby who seemed uninterested and unable to nurse. The lactation consultant asked us to consult on this case. She wondered if we could visit before the mother and baby were discharged and help them see what they had missed. The family was originally from Latin America and although the mother seemed to understand English, the staff was worried that maybe the mother didn't really understand that if she wasn't going to breastfeed, the baby needed to get formula.

> *We sat with the mother, Adora, and asked her about how breastfeeding was going for her and baby Bella, her fourth child. She told us that everything was fine. We asked her if she would show us how she nursed. She brought the hospital bed into a flat position, bunched the pillow under her head, rolled onto her left side, and*

*pulled Bella toward her nipple. Bella gaped and after
Adora moved her onto her left breast, began to nurse.
Bella had a good seal, no dimples, no clicks, and a rocker
motion. Her mouth was open at about 140 degrees, and
her ears wiggled as she nursed. We observed Bella nursing on both breasts, chatted with Adora about her prior
breastfeeding experiences, thanked her for welcoming us,
and left her room.*

We wondered if this was just a simple matter of missed communication as we walked to the nurses' station. There seemed to be a gap
between what had happened with Adora and us, and what had been
going on between Adora and the staff.

When discussing this case with the staff, we found that they
assumed that Adora did not know how to breastfeed and had not been
nursing Bella except when one of them came in to observe a nursing.
When a staff member would "help" Adora with breastfeeding, they
would sit Adora up in bed and put Bella across her mother's lap.
"Adora wasn't very cooperative and Bella mostly was asleep," they
agreed. We told them that Adora had nursed Bella 10 times since the
birth, always lying down. Adora believed that it was wrong to nurse a
baby any way except lying down for the first 40 days. "Why didn't she
tell us that she was nursing when we weren't there?" The answer, "You
didn't ask." This question not asked led the staff to be misled about
what was going on with Adora and Bella. Adora was willing to coop-
erate with the staff, if they wanted her to sit up and hold the baby
across her lap, she was happy to do so. Since Adora didn't nurse for
the staff, they assumed she wasn't nursing at all.

Cheryl & Ellie and Kimberly & Brendan

We had two similar calls from the same local pediatric group within
the space of a few weeks. In both cases the babies were 6 months old
and mostly breastfeeding. The problem for one baby, Ellie, was that
although she had gained appropriately from birth to 4 months she
weighed the same at the 4-month and 6-month weight checks. The
other baby, Brendan, actually lost 3 ounces between 4 and 6 months
after gaining appropriately for the first 4 months.

It's not unusual for breastfed babies to taper off in their weight
gain pattern between 4 and 6 months, especially babies who have had

gained more than 2 pounds a month in the first 3 months. A baby who is born at 7 pounds, for example, and weighs 16 pounds at 4 months, may gain only a pound or 2 in month 5. It is unusual to see a baby with no gain or a loss, so we were concerned, and agreed to evaluate the breastfeeding.

> *The first mother we saw, Cheryl, was the one whose baby, Ellie, had not gained. Ellie nursed well, transferring 3 ounces according to before and after weights on our digital scale, but did not end the feeding herself. We talked for a long time with Cheryl about what had changed in her and Ellie's lives in the past 2 months.*
>
> *We were surprised to learn that she didn't nurse Ellie "after dinner time" and didn't offer the breast again until "breakfast." Cheryl told us that she had been told at the pediatric office that 4 months was time to be sure that the baby wasn't becoming spoiled. "If we don't show Ellie who's in charge now, we'll really have trouble with her later on. I realized that I was giving in to her and nursing whenever she wanted to, even in the evenings and at night. If I don't put my foot down now she'll really be uncontrollable as a teenager. It broke my heart to listen to her cry and cry for me to pick her up and nurse her, but I knew I was doing the best thing for her," Cheryl wept. "Now, I find out she hasn't gained, it wasn't the best thing for her, what have I done?" We were able to help Cheryl understand that she could build back her milk supply if she wanted to nurse Ellie more often, but whatever she decided, Ellie needed to be fed. Cheryl decided to nurse Ellie at least 10 times in 24 hours, and come back for frequent weight checks.*
>
> *A few weeks later Kimberly and Brendan were referred by the same pediatric practice. Brendan had lost 3 ounces between his 4-month weight check and his 6-month weight check. When Kimberly nursed Brendan in our Center, he transferred 4 ounces. Kimberly broke suction to end the feeding; it was obvious to us that Brendan would have nursed longer or on the other breast if his mother had not stopped the nursing. As with Cheryl, we asked about the past 2 months, could she think of anything that had changed, had he begun to sleep through the night, for example.*

"Oh, he sleeps through the night alright. He didn't want to do it at first. The first night he cried for hours. I sat outside his room and just cried, too. But I knew it was for the best, in the long run. I just kept thinking of all the stories on TV, like Columbine and everything. I want him to be a good boy to listen to his father and me. So, I had to start teaching him."

We recognized echoes of what Kimberly had told us in Cheryl's story and asked for more specifics. We asked about what, if anything, made her think about spoiling a 4-month-old baby. She told us that it happened at the pediatric office. One of the ladies talked to her about what to do now that her baby was 4 months old: no nursings after dinner, no nursings until breakfast. The lady told her what the consequences would be if she didn't start teaching Brendan to obey his parents. "She told us that we had to be in charge. It broke my heart but I did it."

A phone call to Cheryl confirmed that it was a woman at the pediatric office who had told her to stop "giving in" to Ellie, the same as Kimberly. We decided to talk with the referring pediatrician about what we had learned. The physician was thoughtful as we explained the advice the mothers had reported receiving at the pediatric office. At the physician's request we described the physical characteristics of "the lady" who had talked to the nursing mothers.

The next week, the pediatrician called us with reassurance that the problem with the office worker in the practice had been resolved. "The lady" was a clerical worker, who had taken it upon herself to give advice to mothers who were breastfeeding.

Here, as with the other cases in this chapter, if we had taken a narrow view of the issue, we would have probably seen many more cases before getting to the real problem. Being open to looking for similarities in cases and patterns in our practice is a responsibility of health care providers. From a medical setting providers should reflect onto the public health sector and vice versa. It's this cross reflection that integrates public health with the medical system and the medical system with public health, making both sectors stronger and more responsive to the health care needs of populations of mothers and babies.

Further Reading

Biancuzzo M. *Breastfeeding the Newborn: Clinical Strategies for Nurses.* 2nd ed. St. Louis: Mosby; 2002.

Cunningham N, Anisfeld E, Casper V, Nozyce M. Infant carrying, breast-feeding and mother infant relations. *The Lancet* 1(8529): 379; 1987.

Lawrence RA, Lawrence RM. *Breastfeeding: A Guide for the Medical Profession.* St. Louis: Mosby Publishers; 1999; Down Syndrome: 477–478.

Righard L, Alade M. Effect of delivery room routines on success of first breastfeeding. *The Lancet.* 336(8723):1105; 1990.

Widstrom AM, Thingstrom-Paulsson J. The position of the tongue during rooting reflexes elicited in newborn infants before the first suckle. *Acta Ped.* 82:281; 1993.

Discussion Questions

1. In the case of the active toddler, Andy, and his new brother, Sam, the suggestion was made that the mother, Kelly, use a sling to keep Sam close to her in a noisy, active house. Do you have experience with slings? Can you think of other problems for which using a sling would be an appropriate intervention?

2. Have you seen a baby self-attach by using the stepping–crawling reflex? In this chapter an assessment of the baby's desire to breastfeed and the baby's ability to self-attach became an intervention. Can you think of other assessment parameters that are also interventions?

Chapter 8

Ghosts

It is the mind that makes the body.

SOJOURNER TRUTH, [SUFFRAGIST, ABOLITIONIST]
(1797–1883)

This chapter explores the role of previous loss and grief in the development of the relationship between parents and their children.

Jennifer, Rob, & Jake

Cristina, a lactation consultant and friend from a midwestern state, called us about Jennifer, a 45-year-old, first-time mother. Cristina had been working with Jennifer and baby Jake for about 4 months, including 1 extended home visit, 2 follow-up office visits, and more than 10 phone calls regarding Jennifer's concerns about inadequate milk, nipple pain, and engorgement. Cristina told us, "I can't understand why she is still concerned. The baby is growing well; mom is pain free, yet she keeps calling me about her worries. I feel that I'm not helping her. When you are in town next week would you meet with her and see if you can help her?" We agreed, and arranged to meet with Jennifer in a private lounge room at a university where we were teaching the following week.

Unlike many mothers with small babies, Jennifer arrived early for her appointment. Well-dressed and groomed, she had a very pleasant, composed demeanor. Curiously, she did not bring Jake with her. When we expressed an interest in meeting him and observing a feeding, she called her partner to arrange for him to bring Jake to her. She stated, "I just needed to get away for a few minutes by myself. I left about four bottles of pumped milk in the fridge for Rob to feed to the baby."

We found comfortable places to sit, poured water all around, and asked Jennifer to tell us about her pregnancy, birth, and breastfeeding experience. She described herself as a latecomer to motherhood; a woman previously focused on her career as the vice president of a large bank. She reported that she knew little about babies before she became a mother. She stated: "Everything went well with the pregnancy. I was nervous, but otherwise fine. The birth—well I'm just glad to be past that. It's just the breastfeeding that is troubling me. I can't get over the feeling that something is wrong—Jake seems uncomfortable sometimes. I find myself waking up and walking the floors at night, worrying about whether or not he's getting enough milk, or if his bowel movements are adequate. Cristina has been very patient with my questions and concerns, but I feel like I'm missing something."

Jennifer reports a lot of anxiety. Could she be experiencing a mood disorder? A thyroid storm?

We asked Jennifer about her physical experience with breastfeeding. While she had experienced painful nipples in the first two weeks, the pain had resolved with the help of her lactation consultant. She said that she was enjoying the firmer, fuller breasts that she had developed, and that she had no physical symptoms from nursing now.

Together we reviewed the referral record Cristina had sent, along with the baby's growth records from his immunization record, which Jennifer had with her. When plotted on a growth grid for breastfed babies,[1] Jake was seen to be

---

[1] Health Education Associates, Sandwich, MA, www.healtheducation.cc.

moving straight along the 75th percentile for weight, 50th for length, 50–75th for weight-to-length, and 90th for head circumference. When asked to describe Jake's behavior, Jennifer replied, "He's not consistent. Sometimes he's content, sometimes he's crabby." On further exploration, Jennifer defined the "crabby" times as lasting for about an hour and occurring every other day or so. She also described his recent tendency to pull away from the breast at the smallest new sound or movement in the room. She decoded this behavior as a sign that he might be ready to wean, and she shared that she was saddened by this thought, as she was not ready to stop nursing.

This report of sadness brought up the opportunity to inquire about her history of mood disorders. Women who were prone to premenstrual syndrome (PMS) and depression may be at greater risk for experiencing postpartum mood disorders.[2]

Jennifer reported that she had no prior history of mood disorders, but had wondered if she might be experiencing postpartum depression. "PMS—yes ma'am! Just ask Rob when you meet him! Poor man. . . ." Because the referral record included no note of Jennifer's physical history, we asked her to fill out a history form with us. Her medical history was largely normal. She was unaware of any thyroid problems and did not identify with some of the thyroid storm symptoms we listed, other than sleep disturbances.

When asked about her reproductive history, Jennifer revealed that she'd had five previous pregnancies, all of which ended in first and second trimester spontaneous abortions. When we expressed our sympathy for these losses, Jennifer began to weep and said, "Rob and I never thought we'd have a baby. We didn't consciously seek this pregnancy, it just happened. I feel like I held my breath through the whole pregnancy. I wanted him so badly, but didn't believe he'd survive pregnancy. Now I barely know how to care for him. Maybe I just wasn't meant to be a mother. I can't seem to do anything right," she continued. "I was scheduled to return to work a

---

[2] Burt VK, Stein K. Epidemiology of depression throughout the female life cycle. *J Clin Psychiatry.* 63 (7):9; 2002.

month ago, but I can't bear the thought of leaving Jake at a day care. I'm so worried and confused."

We sat with Jennifer as she wept, offering tissues, and verbal comfort. When asked what type of help she received with processing her prior losses, Jennifer stated that she had consulted a psychiatrist after the third or fourth miscarriage, and received a few talk therapy sessions and a prescription for sleep medication that she took for a month or so. She stated that she neither sought nor was offered assistance coping with the other losses. "I just climbed into bed and cried for a few days each time. Rob would bring me soup, and rub my feet. I got over it and back to work pretty fast."

Soon Rob arrived carrying an adorable Jake in his arms. An attractive man, apparently in his late forties, Rob was obviously concerned to find Jennifer teary-eyed. He sat down on the couch and unbundled Jake, who had fallen asleep in his car seat. "What's wrong Jen, did Jake chomp on your nipples again?"

"No," she replied. "I'm just so scared."

"Why?" he said, obviously puzzled, making eye contact with each of us in a questioning way. "What's up?"

Jake opened his eyes, saw his mom, and began to express his desire to be with her by fussing, kicking, appearing to try to swim to her through the air. Jennifer reached out her arms, cuddled him, and began to cry again.

"Jennifer has been telling us about the five previous babies she's lost, and sharing her worries about Jake," we explained.

"Honey, those miscarriages were so sad, but they're behind us. Now we have Jake and jeez, just look at him," Rob exclaimed. "He's a bruiser—the pediatrician said she's never seen a better poster child for breastfeeding. You need to stop worrying. Dr. Este assured us that he couldn't be healthier." Jennifer didn't respond, and continued to sob.

At that point, Jake made his desire to nurse known. Jennifer freed her left breast, and competently assisted Jake in latching on in the cradle position. There were no outward signs of maternal or infant discomfort. Jake *latched on with great gusto, suckling quickly for the first minute or so, then settling into a pattern of long, deep suckles interspersed with brief pauses. External attributes of the latch appeared optimal. Suck-to-swallow ratios ranged from 10:1 in the first minute of the feed to 1:1 or 2:1 for the majority of the feeding. Jake's eyes did not leave Jennifer's face, and he appeared to be attempting to soothe her as he massaged her breast with both hands, and worked to make eye contact. As she fed Jake, Jennifer stroked his head and continued to talk about her fears of inadequacy. Rob looked on with both pride and concern visible on his face.*

The amount of shared concern and love was palpable with this small family. Each offered support and comfort to the others by whatever means they had.

We commented on how competently both parents handled the baby, and how responsive they all were with each other. According to both parents, their pediatrician had responded well to their concerns about Jake, and given him several thorough assessments. "She even referred us to an older pediatrician who looked Jake over and agreed that he is a healthy specimen," stated Rob.

We inquired about what type of practical and emotional support the new family was receiving. They reported that both sets of grandparents had taken turns living-in during the first 2 months to help out. Jennifer shared, "They were very helpful and generous with their time, but I couldn't wait for them to leave." Most of their extended family members lived far away. Rob's sister lived in the same town, but he said, "she thinks we're crazy with the breast-feeding stuff. She thinks we should just give Jake a bottle and put him on a schedule. She says all her kids were fed formula, and they turned out fine. She doesn't get it."

Jennifer reported that most of her friends were her coworkers. Some of them had children, but most were older. She had attended a breastfeeding support group a few times, but had been turned off by the presence of older toddlers, one of whom had a green runny nose. She did not want to expose Jake to toddler germs, and

stay home. Her days were filled with caring
…rking out on her home gym, and keeping a
…ke's feeding, stooling, and wetting patterns.
…l about this log, she pulled out a bound,
…n account book and demonstrated how she
…cking facts about his feedings, growth, and
output. "It makes me feel better," she confessed "to see
the number of feedings documented."*

*Together we tallied the number of feedings and dirty dia-
pers over the past 5 days, arriving at a median of 12 feedings (range 10–16) and 4 bowel movements (range 2–6)
per day. We commented on how appropriate this seemed,
and how healthy and responsive Jake looked. Rob
responded with relief, while Jennifer's face hardened. She
took a deep breath and blurted out, "So you're saying
that the only problem is in my head, that I'm just imag-
ining a problem?!"*

*"There's nothing wrong with you, Jen," Rob stated as he
put his arm around her and Jake protectively. Jake
detached from the breast, and began vocalizing to his
mother while he continued to massage her chest and
tried to reach to her face. She closed her bra and pulled
away from Rob, handing Jake to him.*

*We complimented Jennifer on her strong commitment to
having a successful nursing relationship with Jake and
her courage to continue working through her fears. We
summarized, "It sounds like you are having a very hard
time trusting yourself to know what Jake needs, to know
that he will survive. Is that on target?"*

*Tears began to flow again as Jennifer nodded, silently.
Rob began, "Jen, that's silly. There's no one who can care
for Jake better than you. You know so much more than
I do." Jennifer responded, "I know that this doesn't make
sense, Rob. I guess I know in my head that Jake is fine,
that I am doing an OK job. But in my heart . . . well
that's another story."*

During all of these interchanges, we observed Jake's behavior and
found it to be robust and age-appropriate. He appeared to be securely
attached to both parents. His facial expressions mirrored those of his
parents. He "spoke" back to them when they were conversing with

each other. They responded to him by including him in their conversations from time to time. He reacted delightfully to our overtures, but clearly preferred to remain with his parents.

 ## Level 1—History

Findings that stand out include: previous pregnancy losses and initial pain and discomfort with nursing. No striking findings in baby's history with exception of mother's concern about fussiness.

 ## Level 2—Assessment

Nipples are everted; breasts appear rounded with symmetrical veining pattern. Evidence of milk leaking is seen. Baby appears competent in latching and suckling. Long sequences of nutritive sucking and swallowing are observed. Baby's feeding, stooling, and weight-gain patterns and general behavior appear appropriate; baby is reported to meet pediatrician's expectations. Baby is not demonstrating fussy behavior during this visit. Mother and father handle baby responsively and with confidence, which is at odds with mother's contention that she doesn't know how to deal with babies.

 ## Level 3—Symptoms

- Jennifer reports anxiety and fears of incompetence.
- Jennifer has concerns about the adequacy of her milk supply.
- Jake is fussy every other day or so.

 ## Level 4—Problem Formulation

- Jennifer: Discomfort in assuming role of mother, worry about baby, unresolved grief and/or vulnerable child syndrome, and/or postpartum mood disorders.
- Jake: Reported discomfort (unable to assess, not seen).
- Problem of oversupply was considered in conjunction with fussiness, but rejected for lack of daily symptoms (only the symptom of fussiness is noted, but recurrent breast problems; excessive, uncomfortable stooling; and accelerated weight gain in the infant are not noted).

Level 5—Reconcile the History, Assessment, Symptoms, and Problems

History of multiple prior losses via miscarriage indicates ample justification for maternal anxiety. Possible physical reasons for maternal anxiety are not ruled out. History, anthropometric data, assessment, and symptoms do not indicate a problem with milk supply or weight gain.

Level 6—Generate and Prioritize Solutions and Plans for Intervention

There are several theories that address Jennifer's pain. None of these possibilities excludes the others; that is, Jennifer could be experiencing all three of these problems, and possibly more.

The first explanation that came to mind is that Jennifer's unresolved grief and guilt about her past losses has arrested her development through the normally painful stages of adaptation to the mothering role. Daniel Stern has developed a model of the Motherhood Constellation, a group of four psychological themes that mothers encounter as they adapt to motherhood.[3] The four themes and their focus are:

1. Life-growth (her ability to physically sustain the life and growth of her baby)

2. Primary relatedness (her ability to give her baby the love and emotional support it will need to be emotionally healthy)

3. Supporting matrix (her ability to create the support network she and her baby will need)

4. Identity reorganization (transforming her self-identity to give priority to the above activities without losing her core identity)

The life-growth theme is the first and most basic theme encountered by the mother. In this stage, the new mother tackles fears about her ability to keep her baby alive. We have no doubt that Jennifer's previous experience of five fetal losses would have the potential to impede her accomplishment of the life-growth theme. Many women who have experienced such losses blame themselves for the losses, or experience significant loss of trust in their physical, emotional, mental, and spiritual ability to sustain life. This experience can cause the kind of

---

[3] Stern DN. *The Motherhood Constellation: A Unified View of Parent-Infant Psychotherapy*. New York: Basic Books; 1995.

cognitive disconnection Jennifer seems to be experiencing when she talks of her head knowing one thing, but her heart fearing another.

The second possible explanation, that Jake and Jennifer are exhibiting signs of the vulnerable child syndrome, comes from the work of physicians Morris Green and Albert Solnit.[4] These physicians recognized that when children have a difficult or threatening start in life, their parents may come to see them as fragile, magnifying the importance of every physical manifestation and signal from the baby, and looking for malignance in the most benign behavior.

Green and Solnit describe several risk factors for the development of this syndrome, including:

1. *Real or perceived illness in the child*. This could include prematurity, birth defects, hereditary disorders shared by family members, severe or life-threatening illnesses, and medical concerns about the child's health during pregnancy.

2. *Only or last child*. This category includes children born to older parents, parents who have been considered infertile or have experienced pregnancy losses, and children born to parents unable to have future children due to hysterectomy or other conditions.

3. *Psychological issues in the parent*. This may include parents experiencing depression, ambivalent or negative feelings toward the child, unresolved grief or trauma due to prior losses of children or other loved ones, and other psychological reactions to life experiences.

For example, the baby who is placed in intensive care in the first days of life may be perceived to be vulnerable by his parents, who may continue to monitor his breathing, sleeping, and eating habits well into childhood, scanning for something wrong. Again, the loss of five previous babies is a risk factor for development of vulnerable child syndrome.

A third possible explanation arises from Jennifer's suggestion that she may be suffering from postpartum depression or another postpartum mood disorder. The history of prior loss may be a risk factor for this. Another symptom Jennifer describes that may be a hallmark of postpartum depression is pervasive worry. Sleep difficulty, incredibly (almost compulsively) detailed recordkeeping, and persistent concern about Jake's health are other hallmark symptoms.

---

[4] Green M, Solnit AA. Reactions to the threatened loss of a child: A vulnerable child syndrome. *Peds*. 34:58–66; 1964.

In our experience, many problems referred as breastfeeding problems are parenting or personal development issues rather than problems with making and taking milk. In this case, there is a strong possibility that unresolved trauma from prior losses and/or a mood disorder is coloring Jennifer's ability to see the situation clearly, and blocking the growth of self-confidence and trust in her self and her baby. While her partner is supportive, we have worked with other couples where the father has dismissed or amplified the mother's concerns. Family- or couple-oriented therapy can be helpful in elucidating the roots of such concerns and strengthening the couple's communication and coping skills. We therefore planned to suggest that Jennifer and Rob seek counseling to address the anxiety and coping skills, and that Jennifer have a physical to rule out any contributing health factors.

Level 7—Reconcile Prioritized Solutions and Planned Interventions with Problems

The proposed solutions address only Jennifer's anxiety. We add to our proposal a suggestion to maintain a fussiness log to track the pattern of Jake's discomfort, and consult with his pediatrician once a week's log is kept.

Level 8—Evaluate Solutions and Interventions

After we suggested these solutions, we asked Jennifer and Rob for their feedback. Jennifer expressed relief that "what I'm feeling is in the normal realm for women with my history." Rob seemed to feel guilty that he'd been trying to help Jennifer through this by the power of positive thinking, "I feel like I've been belittling your concerns a little, and overlooking how much pain you were in, Jen."

When we asked how Jennifer and Rob would like to go about working on these issues, Jennifer immediately suggested to Rob that she schedule an appointment with a family therapist she knew from her networking group. Rob agreed to this plan. Jennifer also expressed interest in finding a mother's support group that addressed issues beyond breastfeeding. Our colleague Cristina was able to identify some potential group resources. We expressed our intention to share our assessment summary with Cristina and Jake's pediatrician. Jennifer also asked that we send a copy to her midwife. We then all moved toward the parking lot, where we made our farewells.

The Rest of the Story

We talked with Cristina that evening to share our impressions. She was horrified to learn of Jennifer's history of loss. She immediately dug out the chart and found that Jennifer had left the "number of previous pregnancies" slot blank on her history inventory form. We wondered if this was just an oversight, or if skipping over the past was a self-protective mechanism for Jennifer. Cristina felt remiss for missing this large block of Jennifer's history, and immediately connected Jennifer's apparent overreaction to small concerns with her history of loss. We commiserated about those "sleeping giant" issues that complicate many breastfeeding problems. These "giants" may be sleeping, but they cast a large, almost palpable shadow over the situation. They are the kind of things that cause us to think "How did I miss that?" in retrospect.

As we had requested, Cristina contacted us about a month later to update us on this family's progress. She said that Jennifer, Rob, and Jake had been attending family therapy sessions with a therapist who specialized in post-traumatic stress work. In addition, Jennifer was meeting twice weekly with a counselor who specialized in post-partum adjustment disorders. Her physical showed no contributing factors. Jennifer reported that she was beginning to feel more grounded and that her relationship with Rob had improved. She kept a thorough "fussiness" log for a week, but was unable to find any discernible pattern. In consultation with her pediatrician, she and Rob decided that Jake's discomfort was in the normal range. As part of Jennifer's individual therapy, she is writing a paper about her experience that she hopes to publish in a parents' magazine. Jennifer has delayed her return to work indefinitely. She is attending a weekly mother's support group. She reported that she has befriended three other mothers in the group with whom she walks in the park daily, pushing their jog strollers. Jennifer asked Cristina to share with us that breastfeeding continues to give her joy, and that she feels a tiny bit more confident and less worried with every passing day.

Allegra, Todd, & Jordan

Other mothers with whom we have worked remind us of aspects of Jennifer's story.

One is Allegra, a teen mother, who experienced a stillbirth when she was 16. An emancipated minor, she had not intended to become pregnant, but she and her boyfriend were committed to staying together and raising their child. Tragically, their baby died in the ninth month of pregnancy. When we met her after the birth of her second child, Allegra told us openly of her grief at the loss of her first child. She and her boyfriend had broken up in the process of grieving the loss of that baby. Two years later, Allegra and her new partner, Todd, conceived a child. Their daughter, Jordan, was born at 37 weeks' gestation, after an uneventful, healthy pregnancy. Jordan aspirated a bit of meconium and was suctioned and then separated from her parents for approximately 3 hours after birth. When they were united, Allegra put her immediately to her breast, where Jordan licked and nuzzled for the next 2 hours without attaching. Two days later Allegra called for our assistance. Her presenting concern was "I really need breastfeeding to work. My baby is still refusing to nurse most of the time." During our first home visit, Allegra anxiously presented us with a long list of concerns about Jordan's health, nutrition, and her own milk supply, which she read from a notebook she kept by her side. As she expressed her concerns, we observed that Jordan, who was sitting in her car seat across the room, was exhibiting several feeding cues, including mouthing, rooting, and finger and fist sucking. Todd noticed these signs, and tried to call Allegra's attention to the baby. Finally, we interrupted Allegra to ask if she would be willing to offer her breast to the baby. She replied, "It's not time for another feeding. I tried to nurse her only 2 hours ago. I read that you shouldn't nurse more often than every 3 hours, or it spoils babies." Oh, boy!

We asked if she would be willing to experiment with a scientific technique used to assist premature babies in learning how to breastfeed.[5] Allegra's interest was

---

[5] Meyer K, Anderson GC. Using kangaroo care in a clinical setting with fullterm infants having breastfeeding difficulties. *MCN Am J Matern Child Nurs.* 24(4):190–2; 1999.

Tessier R, Cristo M, Velez S, Giron M, de Calume ZF, Ruiz-Palaez JG, Charpak Y, Charpak N. Kangaroo mother care and the bonding hypothesis. *Peds.* 102(2):e17; 1998.

sparked, and she agreed. We then showed her how to perform kangaroo mother care (also known as skin-to-skin). After removing her bra, she tucked Jordan under her shirt. Both mother and baby seemed more relaxed almost instantly. Allegra focused on talking to Jordan and massaging her head and shoulders. Within 10 or 15 minutes, Jordan maneuvered herself into a nursing position, licked a bit, and began to bob her head. "See," Allegra said, tightening her hold on the baby's head, "she doesn't want the breast." We asked Allegra to move her supporting hand down to cradle Jordan's upper back and neck, allowing her room to move her head back. In about 30 seconds, Jordan adjusted her head position, opened her mouth, and attached herself beautifully to Allegra's breast. "Oooh," breathed Allegra and Todd, in unison. "Look at her go!" Todd exclaimed. "Nursing like a champ! She's never done this before." "Wow," said Allegra, "it's like she knows just what to do. We just have to get out of her way!"

We agreed. We observed nutritive sucking patterns, alternating with short bursts of non-nutritive sucking. Jordan released the breast after 10 minutes of sucking, spit up a tiny bit of milk, and maneuvered to the opposite breast, where she fed in a more leisurely fashion for another 10 minutes. The second breastfeeding triggered a voluminous bowel movement. We recommended a same-day weight check with the pediatrician, and unlimited skin-to-skin contact and nursing for the next several days. Both Todd and Allegra seemed receptive to the concept of responding to feeding cues, once the rationale for frequent feeding and the size of the normal newborn stomach was described.

Jordan's demonstration of self-attachment and self-determined feeding made a tremendous difference for Allegra, allowing her to shift her perspective on Jordan from starving victim to capable forager. Allegra called us later that day to announce that Jordan had found her way to the breast 4 more times in the 6 hours since our visit. "She is so smart," Allegra proudly proclaimed, "she can do it on her own, with just a little help from me." Perhaps no one can understand the joy of self-actualized learning like an emancipated teenager!

Allegra reported that she had taken Jordan to the pediatrician the previous day, and that she had gained an adequate amount. She proudly declared that she had burned her list of concerns and questions. Deciphering Jordan's cues had become her focus.

This case forms a powerful counterpoint to Jennifer's story. Despite her past loss, her youth, and relative inexperience, Allegra was able to bridge her fear and self-doubt when she saw a powerful display of her baby's own abilities to seek and sustain nourishment. Rob and all her caregivers were not able to convince Jennifer that her baby had those same abilities, perhaps because her self-concept was at such a low point that she could not see beyond her negative thoughts and fears. Instead, Jennifer followed a path of slowly reassembling her confidence and trust through relationships with others.

Ingrid & Aimée

Ingrid called the Center for help in initiating breastfeeding with her 13-day-old baby, whom she had been formula feeding.

During our home visit, she confided that she had not begun breastfeeding because she intended to give the baby up for adoption. She had not planned to even see her baby after birth, but some instinct drove her to the nursery. Once she saw her little girl, she found that she had to hold her. Two days later she revoked her intention to surrender the baby. She left the hospital with her baby. "Imagine," she told us, "I hadn't planned to bring home a baby. I had no clothes, no diapers, no crib, no toys." Her extended family sprang to action to provide for Ingrid and little Aimée.

Suddenly, on Aimée's 13th day of life, Ingrid was struck with the desire to nurse her. She says, "I wanted to nurse her, but I was afraid that I'd hurt her in some way. I remembered that I had a magnet with a phone number for breastfeeding help on it. I decided to call and see if you could help me."

We suggested that Ingrid place her skin-to-skin, to see what Aimée would do. She had been fed a 3-ounce bottle of formula about an hour prior to our visit, so Ingrid doubted that she would want to nurse. However, within a few minutes, Aimée began to root and explore her mother's chest. Finding the nipple, she licked and suckled a bit. No swallows were heard. We continued to take a history and observe Aimée for the next hour, during which time more nuzzling and licking occurred, but no feeding. Undaunted, we convinced Ingrid to keep Aimée skin-to-skin and rest. We taught Ingrid manual milk expression, and she was able to express a few drops of milk, which we encouraged her to collect and refrigerate in a small container. She agreed to continue to hold Aimée skin-to-skin, and try periodically to express droplets of milk.

When we returned 4 hours later, we found that Ingrid had fed Aimée another 3 ounces of formula after she had been unsuccessful in latching for 2 hours. Ingrid expressed her concern, "She just doesn't seem to get it. I can't let her starve while she's trying." We discussed the possibility of using some expressed milk to tempt Aimée to the breast when she next showed feeding cues. As we sat there observing Aimée, we asked Ingrid to tell us more about her birth and early postpartum experiences.

She began to tell us again how surprising it was to find herself changing her mind about giving Aimée up for adoption. "I hadn't planned to see her, but when I did, something just reached out and grabbed my heart. I couldn't imagine giving her up once I saw her sweet little face. I am worried, though. She won't make eye contact with me—it's almost like she hasn't forgiven me for thinking I could give her up. Is that normal? She can see me, can't she?"

We discussed the focal range of the newborn, and recommended that Ingrid share this concern with the pediatrician at her next visit, or sooner if it continued to worry her.

When asked to tell us more about this concern, Ingrid began to cry, and began to tell us about her first baby, A.J., who died 4 years ago from injuries sustained in a boating accident. Ingrid and her husband took A.J. on a ride on the boat that was their pride and joy. Tragically, their boat was broadsided by another boat whose driver was inebriated. The force of the collision threw A.J. out of his mother's arms and against the floor of the boat. He sustained massive head and spinal cord injuries, which he died from 2 days later. Ingrid, herself uninjured, was severely depressed after his death. She held herself solely accountable for his death. Subsequently, she lost her marriage, her home, and her job. She moved across country, returning to her hometown to make a new life for herself. She never intended to conceive again, believing herself unfit to parent.

One day, she realized that she had not had a menstrual period for a few cycles, and bought a home pregnancy test to verify her nightmare—somehow she had conceived. After much deliberation, Ingrid decided to go through with the pregnancy and give the baby up for adoption. She considered abortion, but found that she couldn't bear to hold herself responsible for the death of another human being. The adoption agency assured her that she could find the baby a good home with a couple suffering from infertility. The baby's father was not a committed partner, and agreed to surrender any rights to the child. Ingrid's family was puzzled, but ultimately supported her decision.

And yet, she decided to keep her baby after all! However, because she had been breastfeeding A.J. during the accident, she couldn't imagine nursing Aimée. As the days passed after discharge, Ingrid found herself increasingly anxious and agitated. Was her apartment clean enough for the baby? Was she doing an adequate job of cleaning and feeding the baby? Each day, she felt more worried about the baby. At her first pediatric visit at 10 days, the doctor pronounced Aimée to be healthy and growing well, yet Ingrid reported that she had feelings of impending doom. On the morning of the 13th day after Ingrid's birth, she awoke feeling hopeful and relieved. As she puzzled over this sudden change in mood, she was struck with the thought that her son had died on his 12th day of life. On some level, she had believed that Aimée would not live any longer than A.J. had. With her joy and relief over Aimée's survival came an overwhelming desire to breastfeed her.

As Ingrid shared this incredible story with us, we noted Aimée's feeding cues were increasing. We encouraged Ingrid to express a few droplets of her milk, which Aimée lapped right up. She still did not demonstrate an urge to latch on to the breast. With Ingrid's permission, we put the precious drops of milk she had expressed in a nursing supplementer, slung it around her neck, and set it to drip a bit. Aimée began to root more vigorously, and suddenly popped herself onto the breast. Almost immediately, she lifted her eyes to her mother's. Ingrid began to sob, "Oh, baby girl, baby girl. Mommy's here." Aimée continued to gaze at her mother, and to suckle sporadically for a few minutes. No sounds of swallowing were heard, but many signs of mother/baby bonding were observed. Aimée detached from the breast after 2 or 3 minutes. We refilled the supplementer with the formula Ingrid had prepared for the next feeding, and showed Ingrid how to use the flow to tempt Aimée back to the breast. Aimée was happy to suckle when the flow was high from the supplementer, being unused to nursing at the breast. Ingrid pronounced herself ecstatic to be nursing her baby. We left them snuggling, with a triumphant mom crowing her news to her family by telephone.

Our follow-up phone calls with Ingrid indicated that she began producing mature milk on the fourth day after our initial visit. After that time she slowly weaned herself off the supplementer, although she continued to give Aimée a feeding or two of formula via bottle daily, "just to be sure." Ingrid and Aimée enjoyed nursing until Aimée was 4 months old, and Ingrid returned to work full time.

Thoughts

Unresolved psychic pain can create or amplify physical sensations and pain. This phenomenon is known as *somatizing*—or creating physical pain from psychological symptoms. In our experience, unresolved psychic pain often is the underlying factor in breastfeeding problems that don't seem to make logical sense, are hard to pin down, or never seem to resolve, but shift to become other problems, as in Jennifer's situation. Whenever we find ourselves banging our heads against the proverbial wall, unable to identify the root or nature of a client's problem, it is helpful to reexamine the problem we are trying to solve: Does it correlate with the reported symptoms and your observations? Often the reported problem is only a surface or somatic representation of the unacknowledged problem(s) that the mother and/or baby are experiencing.

Further Reading

Culley BS, Perrin EC, Chaberski MJ. Parental perceptions of vulnerability of formerly premature infants. *J Pediatr Health Care*. 3(5):237–45; 1989.

Green M, Solnit AA. Reactions to the threatened loss of a child: A vulnerable child syndrome. *Peds*. 34:58–66; 1964.

Kemper KJ, Forsyth BW, McCarthy PL. Persistent perception of vulnerabilty following neonatal jaundice. *Am J Dis Child*. 144(2):238–41; 1990.

Kendall-Tackett K. *The Hidden Feelings of Motherhood: Coping with Stress, Depression, and Burnout*. Oakland, CA: New Harbinger Publications; 2001.

O'Connor ME, Szekely LJ. Frequent breastfeeding and food refusal associated with failure to thrive. A manifestation of the vulnerable child syndrome. *Clin Pediatr*. 40(1):27–33; 2001.

Stern DN. *The Motherhood Constellation: A Unified View of Parent-Infant Psychotherapy*. New York: Basic Books; 1995.

WHO. *Relactation: A review of experience and recommendations for practice*. Geneva: World Health Organization WHO/CHS/CAH/98.14, 1998.

Discussion Questions

1. Jennifer, Allegra, and Ingrid share a history of pregnancy and childbirth losses that colored their experiences of breastfeeding and mothering in different ways. What other types of life experiences could alter how a woman feels about breastfeeding? What effect might these experiences have on the breastfeeding experience?

2. Stern identifies four themes that women wrestle with when they become mothers. Write a question or statement for each theme that is an example of what you might hear from a mother who is struggling with that particular theme.

3. What statements or questions might you hear from a mother who is experiencing vulnerable child syndrome?

4. Many times difficult issues are not expressed in words, but rather in body language, facial expressions, sighs, vocal tone and/or intensity, and other nonverbal communication. Each of us tends to have different skills in picking up on these nonverbal communication methods: some use vision, others hearing, others some other sensory perception to pick up on unspoken concerns and feelings. Ponder your own perceptive process, and try to discern which nonverbal clues are easiest for you to discover. Do you trust your own skills? What can you do to magnify them? What other skills would you like to develop? How could you go about doing that?

Chapter 9

Family Relationships

Among the most disheartening and dangerous of . . . advisors, you will often find those closest to you, your dearest friends, members of your own family, perhaps loving, anxious, and knowing nothing whatever.

—Minnie Maddern Fiske, actress, (1865–1932)

Sometimes solving the breastfeeding problem is the easy part. Sorting out how family relationships are impacting breastfeeding can be much more of a challenge.

Lucy, Wilfred, & Madison

We came to know Lucy during her pregnancy. This was her first baby and Lucy had attended childbirth classes, prenatal yoga, and was getting started at breastfeeding classes at the Center. She couldn't wait for the postpartum belly dancing class, the nursing mothers' group, and the baby singing class. She volunteered at all kinds of jobs, cleaned the meeting room, and picked up toys. Lucy couldn't wait to become a mother. She made lots of friends among the mothers who attended her childbirth class series and planned events as excuses to get together with them on the days in between classes. We expected her to become a regular attender of our postpartum groups. We looked forward to meeting her baby.

> *We learned that Madison had been born at 7 pounds 4 ounces. Lucy called to tell us about how breastfeeding was going (great) how Lucy looked (beautiful) and when we'd see them both (soon). Lucy attended her first nursing mothers group meeting with Madison at 2 weeks' postpartum. Lucy hadn't exaggerated—Madison was beautiful. They didn't come back for the next week's meeting. One of her friends told us that Lucy wanted to be there but something had come up and she couldn't get out of the house. We called, she said that everything was fine, and she'd see us soon. But we didn't see her.*

> *After the next week's group (Madison was now almost a month old) we gave Lucy a call to check in with her. Her voice sounded dull, and although she said that everything was fine, she said it with so little conviction, we knew a home visit was called for. Could we come over to visit this afternoon? We missed her and couldn't wait to see Madison again.*

Lactation care providers, including La Leche Leaders and Peer Counselors, are in an ideal position to refer mothers for evaluation for postpartum mood disorders. There could be many reasons for Lucy's change in behavior, but we needed to make personal contact to find out what was going on.

> *We arrived at Lucy's typical Cape Cod house just after two in the afternoon. She greeted us at her door with a hug and a smile. We chatted for a few minutes in the hall before moving into the living room. Her body posture changed and her shoulders slumped. Her facial expression flattened. She introduced us to her father, Wilfred, who was lounging in the recliner, the side table next to him was covered with piles of used tissues, and over-the-counter remedies for colds, allergies, and GI problems. Two boxes of new tissues completed the array. The TV remote was in his right hand.*

Wilfred rotated the recliner from the direction of the TV over toward us and began to describe his ailments in excruciating detail in a dull monotone. He told us about his sinus problems, his bowel problems, his aches, his pains, his allergies, and his food intolerances. We tried to change the subject to Lucy and Madison but it was almost impossible.

We turned toward Lucy and said "So, tell us about how things are going with Madison." Wilfred broke in before Lucy could respond, telling us how the baby's noises bothered him because of his sinus condition. "Her sounds just reverberate in my head. I just can't tolerate the noise." The TV was blaring in the background. We asked if the TV noise bothered him. "No," was the answer. "The TV is in another sound range from the baby. The baby noises affect my sinuses." He then launched into a detailed description of the lining of his sinuses. We asked politely if his physician had been able to help him. We weren't surprised to learn that he didn't believe in "quacks." "They just want to take parts out of you. My father went to a doctor and that was the end of him. He went to the hospital and died."

Lucy volunteered that Madison was in the back bedroom, we could go there to see her. We got up to follow Lucy when Wilfred began to tell Lucy what he would need before she could leave to go to Madison, including fresh water (the water he had had been out of the refrigerator for too long so it was probably the wrong temperature), some sliced canned peaches, and a sandwich with the crusts removed. Lucy started toward the kitchen when she was stopped by another demand. "Get rid of these used tissues. They make me sick just being around them."

Lucy picked up a trash can from the other side of the recliner and began collecting the used tissues. Wilfred continued listing demands as she crawled around the chair. He now wanted warm water not cold, a specific mug, and a spoonful of honey mixed with vinegar. Lucy finished picking up the tissues, including one that Wilfred dropped to the floor as he was speaking and went into the kitchen. We followed.

Lucy put the kettle onto the stove after first rinsing it out six times. "My father can't tolerate any old water in the kettle. I have to wash it out to get any trace of old water before making his hot water." While the water heated and Lucy rinsed canned sliced peaches from the refrigerator, she told us why we hadn't seen her at group meetings.

"My father retired the week before Madison was born. He wasn't really old enough to retire, it was sort of a layoff from the power plant." As it turned out, Lucy's mother was continuing to work. Wilfred was ill and needed constant tending. Since Lucy was home with a baby, it made sense (to Lucy and her family, certainly not to us) that Lucy take care of her father.

Madison, however, was a problem because her sounds, even her breathing, bothered Wilfred's sinuses. "She sleeps practically all day. She's such a good baby, but of course that means that she's up all night. I'm nursing 10 times in 24 hours, but almost all of them are after my mother picks up my father at around 5:30. Since I can't get out during the day, I have to shop and do all my chores at night and on Saturdays. My mother is so tired from taking care of my father at night that she needs a day to herself, so she brings him over on Sundays, too."

We asked about nursing at night. "Madison sleeps next to my bed and I pick her up whenever she cries. Since she sleeps practically all day I want her to see something besides darkness, so I turn on the lights and sit up to nurse her. Jim has moved into the guest room."

We remembered Jim from childbirth class. Jim had been looking forward to fatherhood with the same enthusiasm as Lucy. They had been together for 5 years before Lucy got pregnant with Madison.

"It sounds like Madison's first month isn't what you planned," we offered. "No," she sighed, "it's been very hard. I'm so tired and so worried about my father, he doesn't seem to be getting any better."

We did determine that Madison had been getting pediatric supervision, that she had gained more than 2 pounds the first month, and that Lucy had no complaints about breastfeeding. We looked in on her and she appeared well nourished and well cared for. We asked if there was anyone in the family who could give her a break from the care taking of her father.

"No, there's just my mother and me now." Lucy paused, "my two sisters aren't speaking to my parents. They think my father should go to the doctor and not take advantage of my mother and me. It was a terrible blow-up. We never really got along, not like other families. My father has always had . . . spells, and well, his health just hasn't been the best." Lucy sniffed as she checked the tea kettle. "My sisters just don't understand."

Lucy went on to tell us about one sister's college gradu-ation. The morning of the June event, Wilfred started worrying about the furnace. "He simply couldn't leave the house to drive up to Boston. My sister was so angry that he didn't come. She hasn't really forgiven him. She's not speaking to me either, she says that I'm foolish to put up with him but really, where else would he go?"

We offered to make some phone calls to find out what kind of com-munity services were available. Wilfred began shouting from the living room. We told Lucy that we hoped to see her soon, that we had been missing her, and that her friends missed her, too.

We contacted professional colleagues and social service providers to find general information about what might be available to give Lucy respite and sent her an envelope full of information. She called to tell us that she had received the information and had discussed some of the options with her parents, but her father refused to consider any-thing except family taking care of him.

"I don't know what to do about Madison. She's starting to be more wakeful and wants to be with me during the daytime. She's not happy staying in the back bedroom while I'm in the living room with my father."

Lucy went on to tell us that Jim also thought that some-thing else should be done besides Madison staying in the back bedroom all day. "He wants me to take care of our baby the way I'm taking care of my father. We have decided to go to counseling. One of the moms from the Center told me about someone who won't mind us bringing Madison to the sessions. I couldn't bear leaving her with a sitter."

Lucy and Jim went to counseling, and before many weeks Lucy and Madison were regularly attending the Tuesday mothers' group and the Wednesday baby singing group.

> *"The counselor helped Jim and I to see that we were enabling my father's illness by not making him go to a doctor. We also realized that we brought Madison into this world and that she was our responsibility first and foremost. We practiced what we would say to my parents and we said it. Not like my sisters. No yelling. But, my mother was still angry with me. She quit her job, and is staying home to take care of my father. Jim and I are still going to counseling."*

Lucy's postpartum experience and her early breastfeeding patterns were controlled by her parents' needs and her feelings of duty to her family of origin.

A new mother is likely to experience some difficulty balancing the roles she plays in her significant relationships and family of origin with her new role as mother to her baby. We can sense that Lucy feels torn between the demands of her recently retired father, her new baby, her husband, her mother, and her sisters. Psychiatrist Daniel Stern's Motherhood Constellation (see Chapter 8) offers insight into the mother's need to transform and reorganize her internal sense of identity.

Stern's fourth theme in the Motherhood Constellation, concerns the mother's need to transform and reorganize her identity.

> *In essence, the new mother must shift her center of identify from daughter to mother, from wife to parent, from careerist to matron, from one generation to the preceding one. . . . This reorganization is an obvious necessity if the mother is indeed going to alter her emotional investments, her allocation of time and energy, and her activities. The new identity as mother, parent, matron, and so on, requires new mental work.[1]*

---

[1] Stern DN. *The Motherhood Constellation: A Unified View of Parent-Infant Psychotherapy.* New York: Basic Books; 1995: p. 180.

Jessica, Arabella, & Trey

There are cases where the baby a woman has envisioned throughout pregnancy is very different from the one to whom she gives birth. This can cause a disconnect between the "dream baby" and the real baby.

One hot and steamy August day we received a call from a local pharmacy. They had provided a rental pump to a mother vacationing in a rural part of the region, but were unable to provide the double pumping kit that she wanted. They wanted to know if we had that particular kit in stock, and if we could get it to the mother, who was staying with family about an hour away from our office. One of us happened to live near the town in question, and offered to take the kit home and get it to the mother over the weekend.

> *We called the mother, Jessica, to make arrangements for a rendezvous. The resulting plan was that she would drop by and pick up the kit on Saturday morning. On Saturday she arrived on time, and came to the door carrying a beautiful two- or three-year-old girl with long brown curly hair.*
>
> *"Hi," she began, "I'm Jessica."*
>
> *"Hi Jessica," we replied, "how are you? And who is this young lady?"*
>
> *"This is Arabella," she said, "my daughter. We've come for the breast pump kit."*
>
> *"Sure. Would you like to come in for a minute?"*
>
> *"Thank you, that would be nice. Wouldn't it Arabella?"*

Jessica settled down on the couch, Arabella on her lap, and began to lovingly comb Arabella's hair with her fingers. We got her a glass of iced tea and a juice box for Arabella who sat quietly, gazing about and taking in the surroundings.

> *"This has been quite a time," she said. "I never thought that having a second child would be so difficult."*
>
> *"Ummm," we replied empathetically, "what has made it difficult?"*
>
> *"Everything," she replied. "I'm really trying to do a good job by the new baby, but the doctor says he's just not growing fast enough. She wants me to get this pump, so*

I can see how much milk I'm making, and so I can stimulate more milk. I don't understand it, I didn't have any trouble nursing Arabella."

"Well," we offered, "babies are very different from each other."

"That's for sure," she interrupted. "Isn't it sweetie! But we do love our baby, don't we Arabella? You're such a good girl."

"Our bodies can change from one baby to another. Has anything changed physically for you?"

"Well, my lactation consultant back home has been over all that stuff with me, you know her, I think—Mary, at St. Lactitia Hospital? She's the one who said that you might be able to provide this pump kit if the pharmacy didn't have it."

"Oh yes, Mary is a great resource. So you and she have been working on this problem together?"

"Yes, she told me she's stumped. She says the baby is sucking well, and that I'm a proven breastfeeder. I just don't get it. It must be him."

"The baby, you mean?"

She nodded affirmatively.

"Can you say more about how he's doing?"

"Well, he's a boy, his father's son—what more can I say. All he wants to do is eat, sleep, and poop. He's pretty grumpy. In fact, he's probably screaming out there right now."

"Oh dear, you mean he's in the car? Let's go get him."

"No, he'll be OK," she replied.

"It's too hot out there—let's move out to the yard so we can be near him in case he needs you."

We carried our drinks out to the yard, where we were able to see the baby still sleeping in his car seat. The windows were rolled down, and the car was parked in the shade. We breathed a sigh of relief, then launched into an infant car safety diatribe.

We then encouraged Jessica to take him out of the car and bring him into the house. She declined this offer, saying that it was her goal to spend all his sleeping time giving special attention to Arabella.

"She's my angel," Jessica whispered, gazing fondly at her daughter who was pursuing a fluffy calico cat across the front door step. "Isn't she gorgeous? We have such a special relationship. I don't want her to be jealous of the time I spend with him. After all, he just needs food, warmth, and diaper changing right now."

There was something about the way that Jessica admired and stroked Arabella that raised concerns in our mind. She was clearly firmly attached to Arabella. Could this possibly be to her baby's detriment? Was she able to see and respond to his feeding cues? Or was Arabella the star of her mothering universe with her baby in a supporting role? How could we gently remind her of the baby's need for attention? How involved should we get in this case? There is another lactation consultant working with mom and baby (although she is several hours away from where the family is vacationing). We have only been asked to provide equipment, not to consult on this case.

"What is your baby's name?" we asked.

"Arabella . . . oh, you mean the new one?" she blushed. "Edward. But we call him Trey, because he's Edward the Third."

"A family name," we replied, "how wonderful. How does Edward let you know when he's hungry?"

"I feed him every 3 hours like clockwork."

"So could you walk us through yesterday? How did the day go, and when did you feed him and change diapers?"

Jessica reported seven breastfeedings, two dirty diapers, and four wet ones during the day.

"And is that a fairly typical day for you?"

"Well, we were on the road for more than 4 hours yesterday, driving here. At home things are a bit different. I have his father give him bottles of formula in the middle of the night so Arabella and I can sleep through. But, while we're here I can't let him cry because he'll wake up my parents—we're staying with them in their retirement home. So last night I nursed him during the night. That was the best feeding we ever had."

"How was that feeding different?"

"Well, he's more hungry, and then it's more relaxed. He's so cute when he grunts and sighs over the milk, you know? He seemed more satisfied after that feeding than any other time."

"Many women tell us that when life is stressful, the nighttime feedings are more rewarding. Maybe you want to consider nursing him during the night feedings, and have your husband give him a bottle of your milk or formula at another time of day, perhaps when you take a nap during the day. Of course, the more you actually nurse, the more quickly your milk supply will increase."

"Hmmm . . . that's a thought," she replied pensively. "I could try that during this vacation, and my mother could feed him while Arabella and I take a nap together in the afternoon."

She then stood up and said, "Well, I'd better hit the road. We have a date with Daddy at the beach, right Arabella?"

We completed the transaction around the pump kit, and invited Jessica to call us or stop by the Center during her stay to check Trey's weight, or sit in on one of our weekly groups. "We'll see," she replied. "Thank you!"

And she rode off into the sunset—never to be heard from again. This is one of the difficulties we have with renting and selling breastfeeding equipment; some women don't seek or want help, just tools. We struggle with the ethics of providing equipment that is not necessarily ideal for the problem. However, it is ultimately the parent's right to choose the solution they think most workable.

Many of the cases that are referred to us for evaluation are made even more complex by the length of time that has gone by before they are sent to us. The more fragile the baby and the more precarious the milk supply when we start to work with a mother and baby, the fewer choices there are in the rehabilitation of breastfeeding. If formula has been introduced before referral to a breastfeeding center, research in Sweden indicates that the chances of breastfeeding continuing are greatly diminished.[2]

—————
[2] Righard L. Early enhancement of successful breast-feeding. *World Health Forum*, 17(1):92; 1996.

Jennifer, Rich, & Rich

One of our local pediatric nurse practitioners, Wendy, was well known to all of the lactation consultants at the Center for her keen ability to identify potential issues before they developed into complex situations. This particular nurse practitioner called one morning and asked if we had time just then for a feeding evaluation of a 2-week-old baby boy who was in her office. She was concerned that something seemed not quite right with breastfeeding, and might be complicated by the mother's diabetes. She wanted to send them right over.

"I'd really like your opinion. The baby checks out OK but the weight gain is marginally low. I don't know if they are just having a hard time getting started or if there is something else going on because of the mom's diabetes. She's been a diabetic since she was a kid and tells me that she's had times of poor control. I also can't tell if she's shy or if she even understands what I'm telling her. I end up talking mostly to the dad. He's the one who seems more 'with it.'"

Jennifer, Rich (the father), and Rich (the baby) arrived later that afternoon. Another man, who was about the parent's same age, accompanied them. This unnamed man sat in the corner, did not make eye contact with us and resisted conversation. We asked Jennifer if she would rather he waited in another room, Rich, the dad, said no, he could stay. We asked Jennifer again and she nodded. "Rich and Rich," we noted, "Is it junior?" "No," Rich answered, "we both have the same name."

We explained that one of the first things we needed to do was to weigh baby Rich. The father was holding the baby and carried him over to the scale. He took off the baby's outdoor clothes and we did a before feeding weight. Jennifer sat on the couch and didn't watch.

Rich carried baby Rich over and sat down again, still holding the baby. Meanwhile, we tried to engage Jennifer in a conversation about her pregnancy, birth, and breastfeeding. She looked to Rich who answered. He explained that, because of Jennifer's diabetes, she had to be careful during her pregnancy, but "nothing bad happened."

Jennifer was induced just after her due date, but after several hours a cesarean was performed. Rich was vague on the reason for the cesarean. "I was just relieved that everything turned out fine." We specifically asked Jennifer about any discomfort she might still be having from the birth. She said she was "fine."

Baby Rich was making sucking sounds and rooting on his blanket where it touched his cheek. As is our practice, we waited to see if the parents recognized the baby's feeding cues. "How do you know when it's time to nurse?" we asked. Jennifer said, "Rich knows. He brings Rich to me." We asked Rich, "How do you know?" He told us that Rich nursed every 3 hours or so, more often if the baby cried and he couldn't get him to stop any other way.

We pointed out the baby's feeding cues to the parents and explained that breastfeeding works best if the baby is fed at the baby's best time. We used a handout to show the parents a variety of cues and pointed out baby Rich's cues to them. Jennifer scooted to the edge of the couch and took the handout, and studied the drawings carefully.

Rich handed the baby to Jennifer and she readied him to nurse on her right breast. She positioned him across her lap in a horizontal position. He latched on and began nursing with a chewing or piston motion. No swallows were observed for the first 3 minutes. We asked Jennifer if she felt any discomfort when nursing. She quietly said no, that she hadn't had any problems. Rich moved his chair closer to Jennifer's right side. His eyes were locked on the baby.

Since we saw little evidence of milk transfer, we wondered if a different position would make a difference.

We asked Jennifer if she always nursed this same way and whether or not this was a typical nursing. She said that yes, it was the way nursing usually felt. Rich broke in, "The feedings are 15 minutes on one side and then I burp him. Then it's 15 minutes on the other side." We explained that the amount a time a nursing takes is less important than the amount of milk the baby transfers. By this time

15 minutes had passed. Rich told Jennifer to end the feeding after checking his watch. She did so by pushing down on her nipple. The baby lunged back at the nipple but Rich took him out of Jennifer's arms and over to the scale. The after weight indicated a change of 00.00.00. No measurable milk transfer, just as we suspected.

Once in a while we are surprised by the difference between our observation of a feeding and the scale report. But in this case, there was nothing about the nursing that indicated that a substantial amount of milk had been transferred, so the scale's numbers correlated with our assessment. We wondered if the baby were in a more upright position if there would be better transfer.

We asked Jennifer if she would be willing to try a different position and she agreed. Sometimes babies are more active nursers if they are more upright. We positioned a thick pillow behind her back, a firm pillow by her side and explained the football position. Rich was still trying to burp baby Rich. We explained that breastfed babies sometimes don't burp. Rich said, "He burps alright, he's a great burper, just like me. Not like Jennifer. She doesn't burp. Ever." Jennifer looked ashamed.

We waited a few more minutes, trying to draw Jennifer out about her diabetes, and discuss her control during breastfeeding. She appeared interested when we talked about the findings that many insulin-dependent, diabetic women feel better and stay in better control while they are breastfeeding.[3] We wondered if that was the case for her. She smiled and said that she thought so, she'd been feeling great. We asked if she had any questions or anything else she'd like to talk about. She said "no," quite firmly.

Rich interrupted telling Jennifer that it was time to nurse on the other side. We worked with Jennifer and the baby to position him in an almost sitting position. We observed chewing motions for the first 2–3 minutes followed by a rocker jaw motion and a 3:1 and 2:1

---

[3] Lawrence RA, Lawrence RM. *Breastfeeding: A Guide for the Medical Profession.* St. Louis: Mosby; 1999, pp. 515–521.

suck to swallow ratio alternating with 12:1. We helped Jennifer and Rich to recognize the difference in sucking and swallowing. Jennifer said that she thought that the baby had done more of the "ear wiggling" nursing a few days ago. We explained that the continuation of the abundant supply that begins on the 3rd or 4th day is dependent on frequent nursings and rapid and thorough milk removal. We described the idea of "supply and demand" and gave her a few pamphlets to read about breastfeeding. In the 15 minutes of nursing, before Rich told Jennifer to stop, the baby transferred 1.8 ounces.

Jennifer seemed interested in the difference in the two nursings and told us that she could feel the difference. We taught the parents how to use the digital scale and sent one home with Jennifer, Rich, Rich, and the unnamed man. They were also given a feeding and stool log to fill out and a suggested ideal volume that Rich should transfer in the next 24 hours. They agreed to return the next day.

Rich immediately began filling out his name and other relevant information on the log. He carried the scale out to the car, then came back in and packed the baby into the car safety seat. When everything was ready, Jennifer and the other man stood up and left with him.

The three adults returned the next day with the baby. According to the log, baby Rich had transferred more than the appropriate amount since the day before. Jennifer seemed more comfortable with us, smiling once and making occasional eye contact, but she still did not volunteer answers, even to questions directed to her. The combined milk transfer after nursing on both breasts was 2.9 ounces, consistent with feedings recorded on the log. In addition, the baby needed a diaper change and we noted a substantial yellow seedy stool and a soaking wet diaper.

We encouraged Jennifer to attend a nursing mothers' meeting, baby singing group, or other offerings at the Center. Rich said that she wouldn't be able to come.

Once again, the pediatric nurse practitioner had identified a crisis in the making. We felt that because of her prompt referral we were able to teach Jennifer and Rich about breastfeeding practices that would support the baby's appropriate growth.

A few days later, Wendy called and thanked us for seeing Rich and his parents. He had gained more than a half ounce per day since her prior weight check. We praised her for her ability to forecast impending crises. Of course we'd be happy to see Jennifer, Rich, and Rich again if the need arose.

> *About 2 weeks later Jennifer called on the warmline at around 4 in the afternoon. Her breasts were hard and full, and they hurt. We asked her when she nursed last. "About 11 this morning." "What's been going on since then? Have you tried to nurse?" "No," Jennifer said, "Rich is at the Bruin's game." We said, "You can nurse without Rich, just pick up the baby and nurse." "I can't. Rich is at the Bruins." "Where is the baby?" we asked, hoping to clarify this confusing conversation. "At the Bruins." "Rich took the baby to the Bruins game?" "Yes, they went to the game, it's a father–son thing to go to hockey games." Jennifer didn't know what Rich was planning to feed the baby at the game.*
>
> *Over the telephone, we taught Jennifer how to hand express into a bowl and reinforced how happy we were that she had contacted us.*

This case is one where the breastfeeding issues are imbedded in family relationship issues. The adult Rich has an inordinate amount of power over Jennifer. The unnamed man also exerted some power over Jennifer. He did not overly participate in conversations, but Jennifer seemed to observe his body language closely. His role in the family was never clarified to us. Jennifer appears to be the classic "woman in silence,"[4] who has not developed her own voice and who seems to have no inner voice that directs her thinking and actions. This type of relationship in which the woman is expected to be silent and the husband has the voice is the norm in some cultures. We also see this dynamic sometimes with teens whose mothers are their voice, the mother answers all the questions, tells us what her daughter likes, when it hurts, and so on.

In our experience, breastfeeding can be an empowering experience for a woman in silence. Breastfeeding may be the first successful

---

[4] Belenky MF, et al. *Women's Ways of Knowing: The Development of Self, Voice, and Mind.* New York: Basic Books; 1986.

activity in the life of a woman in silence. As she watches her baby grow and thrive, knowing that her milk is nourishing the baby, she may appreciate her body and her abilities in a new way. In addition, meeting with other nursing mothers on a regular basis can also be the springboard to individuation. Getting a woman in silence to leave her home can be a hurdle, though. She tends to see herself through the lens of geography, so venturing into strange places can be terrifying.

Later, Jennifer told us that the "Bruins day" was the turning point in her life. She bundled baby Rich up one morning the next week and walked the several miles to the Center for the baby singing group.

> *"It was such a nice day, and being outside with the baby . . . it felt good." Jennifer met other mothers who lived in her neighborhood to go grocery shopping and on adventures together. We learned that she was a professional landscape gardener when she began helping other mothers plan and plant their gardens.*

One of the immeasurable joys of this work is watching the mothers grow as well as the babies.

Further Reading

Belenky MF, Clinchy B, Goldberger N, Tarule J. *Women's Ways of Knowing: The Development of Self, Voice, and Mind.* New York: Basic Books; 1986.

Kendall-Tackett K. *The Hidden Feelings of Motherhood: Coping with Stress, Depression, and Burnout.* Oakland, CA: New Harbinger Publications; 2001.

Discussion Questions

1. Think about what it might be like to be a "woman in silence." Under what conditions might you ask for help? Have you had a client like Jennifer? How were you best able to help her?

2. Lucy wasn't depressed, but 70% of women are reported to experience some type of postpartum mood disorder.[5] How would you handle a referral in your community if you suspected that a breastfeeding mother needed evaluation.

---

[5] Maryland Department of Health and Mental Hygiene. *Postpartum Depression: Incidence, Risk Factors, Diagnosis, Treatment and Resources* 2002. Available at: http://www.4woman.gov/editor/apr02/apr02.htm

3. Using the information presented in one of the case studies in this chapter, complete the eight levels below:

Level 1—History:

Level 2—Assessment:

Level 3—Symptoms:

- _____
- _____
- _____

Level 4—Problem Formulation:

- _____
- _____
- _____

Level 5—Reconcile the History, Assessment, Symptoms, and Problems:

Level 6—Generate and Prioritze Solutions and Plans for Interventions:

- _____
- _____
- _____

Level 7—Reconcile Prioritized Solutions and Planned Interventions with Problems:

Level 8—Evaluate Solutions and Interventions:

Chapter 10

Connecting with Women

A woman under stress is not immediately concerned with finding solutions to her problems but rather seeks relief by expressing herself and being understood.

—JOHN GRAY, FAMILY THERAPIST, AUTHOR
(1952–____)

Sometimes it is difficult to identify the truly therapeutic interaction that takes place during a lactation consult. The orientation of many in this field is focused on physical activities (positioning, latch on, sucking, swallowing, producing, and releasing milk). Many times, feeding problems dwell in the nursing dynamic and can be solved by changes in that realm. Yet, other times we find ourselves at a loss to give a name to the nature of the transaction that alters the mother's experience.

Melanie & Mabel

Melanie called our office for help. "I need help. Breastfeeding isn't going very well." We met with her later that day. "Tell us what brings you here today."

"I'm a wreck about this breastfeeding stuff."

"You're feeling nervous about breastfeeding?"

"Yes, she's my first baby. How will I know if she's getting enough, if she's growing well, if she needs something besides my milk?"

"OK—good questions. Let's take a history, observe a feeding, and talk about those things."

 ## Level 1—History

Indicates full-term, healthy pregnancy. Mother is a primipara. Birth via cesarean, after "failure to progress" for 12 hours. Baby's birthweight: 9 pounds 6 ounces. First mother-baby contact at 6 hours postpartum. Self-attachment at 8 hours postpartum. Breastfed every 3 hours in hospital. Discharged from hospital at 72 hours weighing 8 pounds 15 ounces. Current age 10 days.

 ## Level 2—Assessment

Baby Mabel weighed in at 9 pounds 6 ounces on the Center's scale. She appears healthy and well hydrated. Mother reports an average of 10 feedings in 24 hours since day 4. Daily diaper count: 3 dirty, 6 wet minimum. Mother says her nipples were sore in the hospital, but pain resolved by day 5. No redness or damage is visible. Breasts are small, with everted nipples, and appear symmetrical and even in color and vein patterning.

Feeding observation shows adequate positioning and latch. Minor suggestions: help to increase angle of mouth opening, and reduce mother's shoulder strain.

 ## Level 3—Symptoms

- Maternal concern

 ## Level 4—Problem Formulation

- No problems identified, except self-doubt

Level 5—Reconcile the History, Assessment, Symptoms, and Problems

We reflected on the history, what we observed, the symptom the mother reported, and our inability to identify a problem with Melanie.

> She said, "This would all have been different if my mom were still alive." When asked to tell us more, she tearfully told us of her mother's death 3 years ago. She shared the fresh implications this loss had for her. "How will I learn to mother Mabel without my own mother to help me?"

- New problem identified: Grief over loss and lack of tangible motherly role model.

Level 6—Generate and Prioritze Solutions and Plans for Interventions

We spoke with Melanie for a while about the depth of this loss.

> She said, "I lost my mother before I knew all the questions I should ask her." We agreed that most women feel the need to connect with their mother in a different way after the birth of a child, particularly their first child. Was there another person of her mother's generation in the family who could share some stories about her mother's approach to parenting, we asked? Melanie seemed intrigued by this question, and immediately spoke of her mother's best friend, and an aunt, who both lived in another state. She made plans to contact them within a few days to initiate a discussion. We also discussed the support groups and peer counseling programs available in our area. We invited her to attend a parent/baby singing group at the Center later that week and the breastfeeding group the following week. Melanie seemed cheered by the idea that she had various support options available.

Level 7—Reconcile Prioritized Solutions and Planned Interventions with Problems

Solutions and interventions appear to be reconciled.

Level 8—Evaluate Solutions and Interventions

> *We met with Melanie the following week at the mothers'*
> *group meeting. Her demeanor was light and breezy. She*
> *handled Mabel with much more confidence, exhibiting*
> *an ability to nurse her in three different positions. When*
> *we commented on her skill, she smiled proudly. "Your*
> *visit made so much difference to me. I guess I was feel-*
> *ing embarrassed by my sadness over my mom's death.*
> *Here I have a new baby to take care of, and all I can do*
> *is whine about missing my own mom. You helped me*
> *understand that in a very real way I did lose my mom*
> *again. I never had the chance to absorb her wisdom*
> *about parenting. I need to find some way to replace*
> *that." She then shared her plans to travel to her home-*
> *town, to introduce Mabel to her larger family, and meet*
> *with several of her mother's relatives and friends.*
>
> *"I'm planning to take a tape recorder along so I can store*
> *up some stories about my mom. My grandmother says*
> *that she has several of mom's photo albums and scrap-*
> *books from when we were small. There should be lots of*
> *stuff for me to tap into when I'm missing my mom. I'm*
> *really looking forward to spending some time with my*
> *larger family."*

Entering into parenting causes us to evaluate (consciously or unconsciously) our own parents. How were we parented? What do we think
of the parenting philosophies, methods, and tactics of our own mother
and father? What aspects of their parenting styles do we want to replicate? What aspects do we fear that we will unconsciously replicate?

Research has confirmed the common sense maxim that we typically parent our children the way we were parented.[1] Part of the
process of evaluating our own parents through adult eyes allows us to
reconstruct the narrative of our childhood. If our parents were less
than perfect, can we, as adult children, identify some of the intergenerational trends, social and familial pressures, and other challenges

---

[1] Stern DN. *The Motherhood Constellation: A Unified View of Parent-Infant
Psychotherapy.* New York: Basic Books; 1995, pp. 28–29.

that influenced their behavior? Can we see why they may have made mistakes (even if we can't forgive those mistakes)? This important internal work is completed throughout the early childbearing years.

Stern indicates that the extent to which adults are able to process the parenting they received is directly related to their subsequent ability to form a secure bond with their own children.

> *For example, a new mother could describe her past history with a terrible, inadequate mother, where there is every reason to believe that her mother was, in fact, quite bad. If, however, she has evolved a representation of this unhappy early experience that is coherent, balanced, involving but not overinvolving, she is likely to contribute to a secure attachment pattern on the part of her infant . . . [I]t opens the door for a woman to overcome a bad past or escape the fate of repeating it by way of the psychological work she has accomplished in understanding, putting into perspective, and rendering coherent her past, especially her experience of being mothered."[2]*

When we hear women expressing pain in the memory of their mothers, we find it helpful to listen respectfully, and acknowledge their pain. When her mother is dead, or inaccessible to her psychologically, she must shoulder more of the burden of trying to reconstruct her sense of her own mother within the mothering role.

Hermione & the Triplets

Hermione gave birth to premature triplets after a stressful month on bedrest.

> *Hermione expressed her milk for more than a month before she was able to feed her babies at the breast. The transition to the breast was a slow one, complicated by a bout of mastitis and difficulty pumping enough milk for three babies without the benefit of the stimulation of*

---

[2] Stern, DN. 1995, p. 29.

at-breast nursing. Hermione told us, "Breastfeeding was incredibly important to me, but I was so exhausted that I could feel it slipping away. I was ready to quit before the baby shower." Hermione felt that things changed for her after she dragged herself to a joint baby shower for herself and a dear friend who was expecting a baby. "I could only bear to go because I wanted to support my friend." Yet, she left the shower feeling reinvigorated. She felt hopeful that she could overcome the hurdles in her path, that some day soon her babies would learn how to feed at the breast. Indeed, things changed for her after the shower. Within a week, her babies were solely fed at the breast. Within two weeks, she had a celebratory trip to the waste management center with her bottles, nipples, nipple shields, supplementers, and other detritus of her weeks of toil to maintain a milk supply until her babies could do the work themselves.

What changed? One could certainly argue that the babies reached a developmental stage in that week that enabled them to master the neuromotor tasks of breastfeeding. Yet, if Hermione had not gone to the shower, she believes she would have abandoned breastfeeding within a day or two. So, we ask, what happened at that shower? Did she need to leave her house and babies for a few minutes to get some perspective? Could being in a harmonious, celebratory environment with other women reawaken her faith in herself? Did she receive an unspoken reminder that we are all links in an unbroken chain of strong women who have conceived, birthed, breastfed, and mothered through feast and famine, throughout recorded time? Was it the reminder that she was not alone, that a larger circle of women cared for her? Did she need to reconnect to other aspects of her identity that were temporarily put aside to perform the all-consuming task of birthing and caring for her babies?

Stern writes: "The mother needs to feel surrounded and supported, accompanied, valued, appreciated, instructed, and aided—each to a different degree for different mothers . . . learning to parent is at best an apprenticeship. It is this function that a society of women traditionally fulfilled."[3]

---

[3] Stern DN. 1995, pp. 177–8.

Peer Power

Sometimes the power of other experienced mothers supercedes that of professionals. Two stories come to mind to illustrate the influence of mother-to-mother support.

> *During an infant feeding class in a public health program, we asked women to tell us about the barriers they perceived they would need to overcome in order to breastfeed. One woman spoke up strongly, saying "Breastfeeding is OK for those stay-at-home moms, but it's impossible for working women."*
>
> *Before we could respond, another voice spoke up: "That's not true. I'm working right now, and I'm breastfeeding my baby." Every head turned to the open door of the meeting room. There stood a building employee, broom in hand. "Sorry," she apologized, "but I couldn't help listening in."*
>
> *"Please don't apologize," we replied, "if you have a minute we'd love to hear about your experience."*
>
> *"Sure," she said, continuing to sweep, "what do you want to know?"*
>
> *"How do you do it?" inserted the woman who had made the statement that working women couldn't breastfeed.*
>
> *"It's not that bad. I wake my baby up before I go to work, and we get in a good morning feeding. I learned how to squeeze out my milk, and I do that at lunch and sometimes again during my break. I keep the milk in my lunch cooler. When I get home, the baby is very happy to nurse. He'll nurse a lot during the evening and a couple of times at night. My babysitter gives him the milk from the day before during the day."*
>
> *"Why do you bother?" asked the class participant.*
>
> *"It's really special," answered the worker, "I can't really put it into words, but it's really important to me. I'm glad my baby is getting my milk. It makes me feel better about being away from him during the day."*

We thanked her for the information she shared, and continued with the group. At the end of the group, we asked the participants to tell us whether their infant feeding plans had changed because of information shared, and if so, what made them consider a change. Ten of the 11 participants who entered the room planning to formula feed reported that they now planned to breastfeed. Why? Every one of them mentioned that meeting the working woman was the pivotal moment. Hearing how she managed breastfeeding, and how important it was to her was the key information they mentioned. Subsequent follow-up indicated that 8 of those 11 women did go on to breastfeed; 4 of them breastfed exclusively for longer than 2 months.

The sense of "radar" that women have for others with authentic experience is intriguing. The attention of the entire room shifted to the worker—women who had been inattentive during the group suddenly woke up, physically turned their heads and upper bodies to better see and hear the woman who spoke from her own experience. This is the power of peer counselors. Many research studies have found that trained peer counselors are highly effective in promoting breastfeeding and increasing its duration.[4]

However, one should never attempt to fake this type of interaction. Women can unerringly discern the authenticity of the speaker. The power of these experiences comes from their fresh emergence. It is hard to duplicate this in a planned format. Peer counselors tell us that they find it difficult to continue their work as breastfeeding supporters as their children grow older. The sense of being in the moment with another fades, as time distances one from the lived experience, and revisionist history sets in, their authenticity as peers (being in the same phase of parenting) fades.

Jackie, Jack, & Linda

Another learning experience of this type happened during a mother's support group at the Center. We had been working with Jackie and little Jack for more than 3 months. Jack was a fussy baby, Jackie's fifth

---

[4] Gross SM, Caulfield LE, Bentley ME, Bronner Y, Kessler L, Jensen J, Paige VM. Counseling and motivational videotapes increase duration of breastfeeding in African American WIC particicpants who initiate breast-feeding. *J Am Diet Assoc.* 98(2):143–8; 1998.

Martens PJ. Increasing breastfeeding initiation and duration at a community level: An evaluation of Sagkeeng First Nation's community health nurse and peer counselor programs. *J Hum Lact.* 18(3):236–46; 2002.

Merewood A, Philipp BL. Peer counselors for breastfeeding mothers in the hospital setting: Trials, training, tributes and tribulations. *J Hum Lact.* 19(1):72–6; 2003.

baby. She had nursed all of her children, now ranging from 2 to 13 years old. Jackie was herself a powerful voice, offering guidance and information to others attending the support group. She never missed a group meeting. Many group participants deferred all authority to Jackie, because she had successfully nursed and mothered so many children.

Numerous consults had resulted in solutions that reduced, but did not alleviate Jack's feeding discomfort. He spit up, sometimes repeatedly, after each feeding. He was fussy after every feed, apparently experiencing a good amount of gastric distress.

Jack's pediatrician was unable to find any organic causes for his difficulties. We had suggested a few times that Jackie try eliminating cow's milk from her diet.[5] She did not act on this suggestion, saying he was apparently just a cranky baby. Eventually, little Jack became symptomatic with eczema—red, dry patches blooming on his cheeks, in the folds of his elbows, and elsewhere. His discomfort became more marked.

> *One day Linda, a mother who was new to support group, spoke up about her experience with cow's milk intolerance. She told of the remarkable change in her baby when she had been on a dairy-free diet for 10 days. Jackie's ears perked up. "Really," she said, "how interesting—tell me more!" Jackie called us later that day to talk about a dairy-free diet. We asked if she still had the written information we had given her on at least two occasions. "Sorry," she said, "I didn't keep it. I thought you were just trying to give me excuses for his crabbiness. I really didn't realize that this could be a real problem until I heard Linda mention it."*

We cannot underestimate the influence and importance of supportive peers. The vast majority of successful community breastfeeding support programs have strong components of mother-to-mother or peer support. The support needs of new mothers are so varied and unique that it is

---

[5] Arshad SH. Food allergen avoidance in primary prevention of food allergy. *Allergy.* 56 Supp/67:113–6; 2001.

Restani P, Gaiaschi A, Plebani A, Beretta B, Velona T, Cavagni G, Poiesi C, Ugazio AG, Galli CL. Evaluation of the presence of bovine proteins in human milk as a possible cause of allergic symptoms in breast-fed children. *Ann Allergy Asthma Immunol.* 84(3):353–60; 2000.

Saarinen KM, Juntunen-Backman K, Jarvenpaa AL, Klemetti P, Kuitunen P, Lope L, Renlund M, Siivola M, Vaarala O, Savilahti E. Breast-feeding and the development of cows' milk protein allergy. *Adv Exp Med Biol.* 478:121–30; 2000.

really not possible for an individual or small group of individuals to meet them. We are struck with the jarring contrast between Stern's envisioned support matrix, the creation each mother is supposed to weave to fully support her baby, and our image of the reality of most new mothers, ensconced in their individual (often lonely) households, usually barely connected to spotty support from their family, community, or health care system. Additionally, there is little universal knowledge about breast-feeding disseminated throughout culture. Breastfeeding education is rarely offered to the general public, and only cursorily to prospective mothers. What is the breastfeeding knowledge of a new mother's support matrix? Childbearing women of today may or may not have been breast-fed themselves. The child health knowledge one's own mother carries is assumed by modern culture to be largely outdated; witness the debacles many families have experienced over safe infant sleep positions. When their own children were small, today's grandmothers were told to place them on their stomachs for sleep, that they might choke on their spit-up if they were placed on their backs. Yet today, for good reason, "back to sleep" is the motto of the land. We are facing an epidemic of babies with misshapen heads because parents are so afraid to lay their babies on their stomachs at all. Grandmothers bite their tongues to keep from sug-gesting placing babies on their tummies to play. This does not engender a climate of shared knowledge and wisdom.

What results is that the mother takes more seriously upon herself the safe negotiation of the life-growth theme of the Motherhood Constellation. More and more responsibility rests on her to ensure the safety and health of her baby. What mothers need is a larger, trusted support matrix. A place to receive valid information and support, to feel connected, part of the tribe, part of humankind and not an anomaly—a nursing mother, single-handedly performing miracles in her living room, alone.

Amber, Mrs S., & Tariq

We made a home visit to one young mother, Amber, who told us on the telephone that her 5-day-old son Tariq had not yet nursed at the breast. We arrived at her apartment to find Amber's grandmother giving Tariq a bottle of expressed milk, while Amber collected milk for the next feeding with her small battery-operated pump. Amber's grandmother, Mrs S., clearly enjoyed her interaction with her small great-grandchild. She told us, "I didn't breastfeed myself—times were different when I had my babies—but I think it's good for him, and his mama, as long as she gives him enough milk and it doesn't wear her out."

Level 1—History

Amber is 17 years old and lives with her grandmother. Her boyfriend, Tariq's father, "comes around sometimes." She is estranged from her parents, and is on a month long leave from high school. Her pregnancy was reportedly healthy, although she didn't begin prenatal care until the fifth month. She delivered Tariq at 41 weeks' gestation, after a 15-hour "intense" labor. She had an epidural 2 hours before the birth. Tariq was born at 7 pounds 8 ounces.

> *She told us: "When he was about an hour old, they put him on me and he looked me right in the eye, and then scooted over to my nipple. He licked it and stuff, but didn't suck. After another hour, I was getting really worried. The nurse said he'd be OK, then she came over and grabbed my boob in one hand, and his head in the other. She basically crammed it into his mouth. He didn't like that, I'll tell you. He started to scream. Finally they took him away and gave him some sugar water. After that, he freaked out every time I put him near the breast. I started pumping in the hospital, and made them give him that in a bottle. They wanted to give him formula, but I said 'No way!' I think it's garbage.'"*

> *"Since we got home from the hospital, I've tried him on the breast several times. I even tried not to feed him for several hours to see if he'd take it when he got really hungry, but he won't."*

His discharge weight was 7 pounds 2 ounces. First pediatric follow-up is scheduled in 2 days.

Level 2—Assessment

We observed both of Amber's breasts as she pumped. Prior to pumping, they appear well rounded, symmetrical. Her nipples are on the flat side, and are large in diameter. The pump easily drew out a good amount of breast and nipple tissue; after the pumping session, her nipples reverted to a flat appearance. Pumped volume was observed at 2 ounces on the right breast, 1.5 on the left (an average pump yield according to Amber). She reported that she had been pumping 6–7 times daily, with an average daily yield of 18–22 ounces. We applauded her hard work and commented loudly on the abundance of her milk so that her grandmother overheard it.

Tariq appeared well hydrated and healthy. He suckled vigorously at the bottle, transferring 1.5 ounces in less than 5 minutes. (He had already taken 1 ounce or more prior to our arrival.) We complimented Mrs. S on the cradled, nursing-like position she held him in. Amber reported a minimum of four yellow, seedy bowel movements daily. We estimated his nutrient needs to be 18.75 ounces daily (7.5 pounds × 2.5 ounces/pound)—he was reportedly taking between 18 and 20 ounces of expressed milk by bottle.

> *We inquired about Amber's long-term breastfeeding goals, and she replied that she'd like to nurse him for at least a year. She'll be returning to school in 4 weeks, but plans to take her pump along with her. Mrs. S, who is retired, will be caring for Tariq during school hours. She summarized, "I'm already good at pumping milk, but I want to get breastfeeding down. I want to feed him myself."*

Level 3—Symptoms

Baby refuses to feed at breast

Level 4—Problem Formulation

- Refusal to feed related to force applied at first feeding?[6]
- Delay in feeding due to epidural?[7]
- Possible nipple preference (mother's flatish nipple versus firm bottle teat)

---

[6] Widstrom AM, Thingstrom-Paulsson J. The position of the tongue during rooting reflexes elicited in newborn infants before the first suckle. *Acta Paediatr*. 82(3):281–3; 1993.

[7] Baumgardner DJ, Muehl P, Fischer M, Pirbbenow B. Effect of labor epidural anesthesia on breast-feeding of healthy full-term newborns delivered vaginally. *J Am Board Fam Pract*. 16(1):7–13; 2003.

Hildebrandt HM. Maternal perception of lactogenesis time: A clinical report. *J Hum Lact*. 15(4):317–23; 1999.

Ransjo-Arvidson AB, Matthiesen AS, Lilja G, Nissen E, Widstrom AM, Uvnas-Moberg K. Maternal analgesia during labor disturbs newborn behavior: Effects on breastfeeding, temperature, and crying. *Birth*. 28(1):5–12; 2001.

Level 5—Reconcile the History, Assessment, Symptoms and Problems

History did not reveal any other contributing symptoms or possible problems, but further pediatric evaluation could be needed.

Level 6—Generate and Prioritze Solutions and Plans for Interventions

- Observe a feeding attempt
- Identify problems and develop interim plan for moving feeding to the breast
- Refer baby to pediatrician for further work-up

Level 7—Reconcile Prioritized Solutions and Planned Interventions with Problems

> *We asked Amber if she would show us what happens when she tries to feed Tariq. She agreed. He had finished the bottle. Amber scooped him up from Mrs. S's arms, and changed his diaper. We observed a 3-inch circle of yellow, seedy stool in his diaper, along with a healing circumcision. She asked us to watch him for a minute while she washed her hands. She then picked him up, carried him to the couch, lifted her T-shirt and pulled a sports bra up over her breast. We encouraged her to stop for a minute, and take the sports bra completely off, keeping the T-shirt on for warmth.*

We were concerned by the amount of pressure the sports bra was applying to her breast. It was indenting the breast so deeply, that it changed the angle at which the breast hung by about 40°, moving her nipple from the level of the baby's mouth to his eyebrow.

> *Through all these changes, Tariq seemed content to gaze at his mother. Once she had removed her bra and settled back into her seat, we moved over to sit beside her so we could observe the latching process in detail. She chose to try to feed him at her left breast in the cradle position. We watched her body language and his as she brought Tariq in closer for the feeding. He lay quietly in her arms until*

he saw the breast, then his body posture stiffened. When he stiffened, her shoulders raised, and she began to become tense. She moved the forearm on which he was laying tightly into her body. He responded by arching and pulling away, squawking.

"See," she sighed, "he just won't do it."

It takes lots of practice to learn a new skill," we replied, "let's try something a little different."

We asked her to switch her hand positions around so that her right hand supported his body weight, with her palm resting on his upper back and neck. Her left hand could cup the breast if needed. With some coaching, she raised him to the breast, watching for his mouth to open. Although his mouth was open when he was away from the breast, complaining mildly, he sealed his lips firmly shut when she raised him to the nipple. Undaunted, we asked her to hand express a droplet of milk, and try again. When she raised him to the breast the second time, he stuck out his tongue and tasted the milk, but didn't open his mouth. After a minute, we asked her to move him away again. As she lifted him back to the nipple, he opened his mouth to about 120° and latched on. Amber was amazed, "Oh my gosh! He's nursing!" Sure enough, Tariq suckled at a 10:1 pattern for about 30 seconds, shifting quickly to a 2:1 pattern within the first minute.

"Look, Grandma," she cried, "my baby sucks!"

We all had a good chuckle, while we watched Tariq and Amber's obvious enjoyment of nursing.

⑧ Level 8—Evaluate Solutions and Interventions

Tariq continued to suckle at the breast for another 10 minutes, while we wrapped up our consult.

"This is so awesome," Amber said, "thank you so much for coming over."

We left her with a plan to continue putting him to the breast every time feeding cues were observed, and to continue to pump for a few minutes after each feeding to ensure that milk removal was optimal while he became accustomed to nursing at the breast.

> *She called us later that day, to tell us that Tariq had nursed 3 times in the 6 hours since our visit. "Now he that he's figured it out, he doesn't want to stop nursing." She was very pleased with their progress.*
>
> *Two days later she called to tell us that Tariq's doctor had pronounced him a "butterball," as he weighed in at 7 pounds 10 ounces, up 8 ounces from his discharge 5 days ago. She thanked us again for coming by, and said that she wanted to know what magic we used to get Tariq to nurse. "You and Tariq were the magical ones," we replied. "You just needed a little coaching to get him going." "Nope," she denied, "it has nothing to do with that positioning thing. I can hold him any way I want now, and he'll nurse, no problem. I think the magic happened when you sat down on that couch with me. I suddenly thought, 'I can do this.' It was like a psychic transfer from you to me. Suddenly I just knew I could do it."*

Daniel Stern writes, "the mother needs and wants to be 'held,' valued, appreciated, aided, and given structure by a benign, more experienced woman who is unequivocally on her side."[8] This may be one of the "secrets" of the lactation consultant: her womanly presence.

Many women long to be seen, heard, and accepted. When we listen respectfully, welcome her words and descriptions, and accept her right where she is in the moment, it may allow her to make changes in how she sees, feels, understands, and reacts to her situation. Sadly, many women grow to maturity without having received adequate respect and/or acceptance. Respectful listening and inquiry is in itself a great gift to many new mothers.

The ultimate goal of the staff and faculty of the Center is to help mothers and fathers to fall in love with their babies, and integrate them into a healthy family structure. This goal takes precedence over method of feeding, because love is a more basic need than type of

---

[8] Stern DN. 1995, p. 183.

food. We acknowledge the work of our esteemed colleagues, who clarified for us that oxytocin is the hormone of love.[9] One of the best gifts we could imagine for the children of the world is that they are cared for by parents who are high on oxytocin, the hormone of love.

Further Reading

Gladwell M. *The Tipping Point: How Little Things Can Make A Big Difference.* New York: Back Bay Books; 2002.

Jordan JV, Kaplan AG, Miller JB, Stiver IP, Surrey JL. *Women's Growth in Connection: Writings from the Stone Center.* New York: The Guilford Press; 1991.

Odent M. *The Scientification of Love.* London: Free Association Books; 1999.

Stern D, Bruschweiler-Stern N, Freeland A. Special Needs: Premature or Handicapped Babies, In: *The Birth of a Mother: How the Motherhood Experience Changes You Forever.* New York: Basic Books; 1998, pp. 181–201.

Discussion Questions

1. Tariq and Amber had difficulty getting breastfeeding started. What strategies have you found effective in such cases? In this case, skin-to-skin contact seems to have jump-started Tariq's drive to breastfeed. What possible benefits and risks can you identify for skin-to-skin care? What are the potential benefits and risks of other strategies you might suggest?

2. What is your reaction to the philosophy that for babies "love is more important than type of nutrition?" Explore your reaction and how it affects your work with parents who choose different feeding methods.

3. Hermione struggled to maintain her milk supply before her premature triplets were physically able to nurse at the breast. What other strategies can be used to build and maintain milk supply when the mother is dependent on pumping for milk production? What are the risks and benefits of each strategy?

[9] Nissen E, Gustavsson P, Widstrom AM, Uvnas-Moberg K. Oxytocin, prolactin, milk production and their relationship with personality traits in women after vaginal delivery or cesarean section. *J Psychosom Obstet Gynaecol.* 19(1):49–58; 1998.

Uvnas-Moberg K, Eriksson M. Breastfeeding: Physiological, endocrine and behavioural adaptations caused by oxytocin and local neurogenic activity in the nipple and mammary gland. *Acta Paediatr.* 85(5):525–30; 1996.

The First Epilogue

Imagine women cooking together. An extended family, grandmothers, aunts, mothers, daughters, sisters, and cousins: An intergenerational melange is needed to feed an enormous family. Auntie prepares her special spices for a sauce. Mother grinds the grain. Older sister prepares vegetables. The younger children fetch water. You are ten years old. Your task is to keep the babies safe, to watch the toddlers and sleeping babies. You are sitting near the older girls and women, but not yet part of their inner circle. You are not a child relegated to fetching and carrying. Your eyes are on the babies and toddlers, but your ears are with the nearby women who talk of women's things: birth and marriage, breastfeeding and weaning. Some of the stories you have heard many times. You pull closer when the women lower their voices. You strain to hear what happened when the baby wouldn't nurse, about the mother who didn't have enough milk. You learn why these things happen, and how the problems were solved . . .

Breastfeeding is natural. Lactation progresses normally after childbirth, yet the process is enhanced by skill and knowledge. It is not enough that the mother desires to breastfeed. It is not enough that she is knowledgeable about breastfeeding.[1] The mother must be helped to breastfeed;[2] more help means greater chance of success.

---

[1] Ertem IO, Votto N, Leventhal JM. The timing and predictors of the early termination of breastfeeding. *Pediatrics*. 2001;107(3):543–508.

[2] Morrow AL, Guerrero ML, Shults J, et al. Efficacy of home-based peer counselling to promote exclusive breastfeeding: A randomised controlled trial. *Lancet*. 1999; 353(9160):1226–1231.

We speculate that our great-grandmothers seamlessly integrated their support of breastfeeding mothers and babies into their daily lives. Girls observed younger siblings at the breast. Women told each other cautionary tales of breastfeeding problems and successes.

As we search through the writings of generations past, we find scant reference to breastfeeding and human milk, perhaps because nurturing babies and young children at the breast was expected, normal, and appropriate. The oral tradition of women's knowledge related to breast-feeding has not been preserved in many families, in many cultures. Perhaps the very ordinariness of breastfeeding contributed to the decline in the initiation and duration rates we have seen in modern times. Like hemlines, how to feed babies has been subject to the whimsy of fad and fashion. As the "fashion" winds shifted to formula and bottles, women's knowledge of how to help women breastfeed has been distorted or lost.

It is our belief that we have not only lost breastfeeding as the cultural norm, we have lost the stories that women shared with each other, the stories that provided the matrix of knowledge and support that enabled breastfeeding from one generation to another. As clinicians and educators we see ourselves and our next generation bridging the gap from a time in the past when breastfeeding was the cultural norm, to a time in the future when breastfeeding babies and young children will be the norm again.

All over the world, caring individuals have chosen to dedicate themselves to the work of reclaiming breastfeeding as a baby's birthright, a mother's joy, and a family's pride. They have wondered how something so pleasurable and natural as breastfeeding, so biologically appropriate and species-specific as human milk could need advocates, supporters, boosters, protectors, and dedicated clinicians in this modern age. They have begun to tell each other the stories and cautionary tales, to reclaim this lost piece of women's knowledge.

It has been our honor to be part of this process as educators of thousands of health care providers, mother-to-mother supporters, counselors, educators, and consultants. It has been our privilege to be part of this process as clinicians working with mothers and babies in a variety of settings.

The case studies we have shared in this work are our professional guideposts, the cases we often recount with each other, and find ourselves telling and retelling in training programs. It is our belief that encoded in the stories of these families are some of the keys to understanding the deeper process and meaning of lactation counseling. It is our sincere hope that these case studies will be of assistance to you, the reader, in your quest to provide the best possible support for the families you serve.

Glossary

A

Acidophilus: A type of helpful bacteria that provides an acidic environment in the gut (which discourages overgrowth of unhelpful microbes).

Affect: Facial expression.

Alternate massage: Massaging and compressing the breast when the baby pauses between suckles while nursing.

Anoxic event: A period of time when breathing does not occur, resulting in temporary oxygen depletion.

Anthropometric: Weight and height data.

At-breast supplementer: A feeding tube device used to deliver expressed milk or formula while the baby feeds at the breast.

C

***Candida albicans*:** A pseudo-fungal organism that normally resides on mucous membranes, but can become overgrown when the immune system is suppressed.

***Candidiasis*:** Overgrowth with *Candida.*

Celiac disease: A sensitivity to gliadin, a component of gluten, a protein found in wheat and other grains. In affected individuals, gliadin damages the villi of the small intestines and results in diarrhea, weight loss, or growth faltering, gastrointestinal discomfort and abnormal stools.

Cesarean: Surgical birth, removal of the baby by incision through the abdomen into the uterus.

D

Down's Syndrome: A congenital genetic disorder causing mental retardation, low musle tone, and short stature.

E

Eczema: A skin rash with small, itchy red or white bumps that is often a symptom of allergy.

Emancipated minor: A person under 18 years of age who has been released from parental control and supervision through a legal proceeding.

Excoriated: Abraded; skin broken; scratched or rubbed off.

Engorgement: Swelling in the lactating breast caused by increased blood and lymph flow and/or excess milk storage due to ineffective or infrequent milk removal.

Everted: Standing out or sticking out from the surface.

G

Gastric Bypass Surgery: A surgical procedure that reduces the size of the stomach by stapling the lower stomach and connecting the small intestine to the much smaller remaining upper stomach tissue. This procedure is done to promote weight loss.

Gastroenterology: The medical specialty that is concerned with the health of the gastrointestinal tract.

Gastrointestinal: The digestive system, including the stomach, small and large intestines, colon, and rectum.

Gestation: Growth.

Gestational diabetes: A type of diabetes that arises during, and is limited to, pregnancy.

Grand Multipara: A woman who has had more than five babies.

H

Hyperbilirubinemia: An excess of bilirubin (a breakdown product of red blood cells) in the blood. One symptom of hyperbilirubinemia is jaundice, or the yellowing of the skin.

I

Inflammation: A process of swelling in the spaces between cells, often triggered by the presence of substances (e.g., reabsorbed milk from over-full milk-making cells) that the body perceives to be foreign.

Inverted: Drawn inward.

J

Jaundice: A symptom of hyperbilirubinemia that is the yellowing of the skin and the whites of the eye.

K

Kangaroo Mother Care: Use of skin-to-skin care for premature infants.

L

Lochia: Normal uterine discharge after birth consisting of blood and tissue. Lochia rubra is red; Lochia serous is creamy yellow in color.

M

Mastitis: Inflammation of the breast created by infective or noninfective causes.

N

Neuralgia: Pain from nerve inflammation or trauma.

Neurohormonal: Integration of the nervous and endocrine system.

Neurologic: Pertaining to the nerves and nervous system.

Neuromotor: Integration of the nervous and muscular systems.

NICU: Neonatal intensive care unit, hospital unit where preterm and ill infants are treated. Also called special care unit (SCU) in some facilities.

Nipple shield: A thin silicone, latex, or rubber device placed over the surface of the nipple and breast during feedings.

Nonnutritive pattern: High ratio of suckling to swallowing (> 3:1) that indicates that milk transfer is insignificant.

Nutritive pattern: Low ratio of suckling to swallowing (1:1, 2:1) that indicates that milk transfer is significant.

O

Oxytocin: The hormone that causes the contraction of the cells around the alveoli, forcing the milk down the ducts toward the nipple.

P

Palliative: Comforting.

Peripartum: Around the time of the birth.

Postpartum: After the time of the birth.

Prematurity: Birth of a baby before 38 weeks' gestation.

Prenatal: During the pregnancy.

Primipara: A first-time mother.

Psoriasis: A chronic skin disease characterized by small red papules covered by fine white scales.

Psychic: Relating to the human mind and emotions.

R

Raynaud's phenomenon: Temporary compromised blood flow precipitated by cold that results in extreme pain and blanching (whitening) in the fingers, toes, and occasionally the nipples.

REM sleep: Sleep state characterized by Rapid Eye Movement, which indicates that the baby is in a light sleep state.

S

Satiety: Fullness, satisfaction.

Self-attachment: The infant's demonstrated ability to find and attach to the breast using the stepping–crawling reflex.

SIDS: Sudden Infant Death Syndrome; death in a child under 1 year of age caused by cessation of breathing.

Somatic: Pertaining to the body and bodily symptoms.

Somatize: To express emotional discomfort through physical symptoms.

Spontaneous abortion: A miscarriage, and unintended end to pregnancy.

Suck/swallow: Ratio of audible sucks to swallows.

Symmetrical: Appearing to be about the same size and appearance.

Symptomology: Collection of symptoms or complaints about the situation.

T

Therapeutic: Effecting change.

Thrush: An oral overgrowth of *Candida*.

Thyroid Storm: A potentially life-threatening episode of overproduction of thyroid hormones. Symptoms include extreme agitation, rapid weight loss, inability to sleep, racing pulse, and sensation of being overheated.

V

Vector: An agent or item that transfers material from one place to another.

Vulnerable child syndrome: The perception that a child is fragile, which may arise when a child has a difficult or threatening start in life. This syndrome may lead parents to obsess about the child's health, magnifying the importance of every physical manifestation and signal from the baby, and looking for malignance in the most benign behavior.

Y

Yeast: A short name for *Candida* or other similar fungi.

Index

About the Authors

Karin Cadwell, PhD, RN, IBCLC is a nationally and internationally recognized speaker, researcher, and educator. She convened Baby-Friendly USA, implementing the WHO/UNICEF Baby-Friendly Hospital Initiative in the U.S., is a delegate to the U.S. Breastfeeding Committee and the USDA's Breastfeeding Promotion Consortium, and was visiting professor and program chair of the Health Communications masters degree at Emerson College and is an adjunct professor at the Union Institute and University.

Karin served on the IBLCE Panel of Experts to develop the first certification exam for International Board Certified Lactation Consultants (IBCLC). She is the author of numerous books and articles including *Maternal & Infant Assessment for Breastfeeding and Human Lactation* and *Reclaiming Breastfeeding for the US*, was awarded the designation IBCLC in 1985 for "significant contribution to the field," and has since been recertified by exam.

Cindy Turner-Maffei, MA, IBCLC is national coordinator of Baby-Friendly USA, implementing the WHO/UNICEF Baby-Friendly Hospital Initiative in the U.S.. She has extensive experience as a nutritionist and breastfeeding educator in WIC and other public health programs. Cindy is a member of breastfeeding coalitions on the local, state, and national levels, and serves as a delegate to the U.S. Breastfeeding Committee and the USDA's Breastfeeding Promotion Consortium.

Cindy is also an adjunct professor at the Union Institute and University. She is an author of *Maternal & Infant Assessment for Breastfeeding and Human Lactation* and *Reclaiming Breastfeeding for the US*, as well as the La Leche League International Independent Study Module *Strategies for the Implementation of the BFHI in the United States*.

Karin and Cindy are faculty members of The Healthy Children Project and teach in the Lactation Consultant concentration at the bachelor's, master's, and Ph.D. programs at Union Institute and University. They are also lactation consultants in East Sandwich, MA (USA) at *the Center for Breastfeeding*.

Karin Cadwell and Cindy Turner-Maffei can be reached at *thecenter@healthychildren.cc*.